Weight Loss Surgery: The Essential Guide

Bilal Alkhaffaf

A comprehensive illustrated guide to understanding obesity, choosing weight loss treatments, and life after surgery.

First Edition 2023

Copyright Statement

Who is this book for?

This book is aimed at anyone who, despite significant efforts, has struggled with their weight and is exploring other tools including surgery to help them gain back control. It is also useful for anyone who has already undergone surgery, as they navigate through their post-operative journey and the longer-term challenges that may arise. The sheer volume of information available online means that it is often challenging to know where to start and what to believe, and so this book aims to provide the most up-to-date, reliable information from a reputable and experienced source. The topics are based on common questions which our patients have asked of our team over the years.

In addition, this guide will benefit friends and families of anyone considering weight loss surgery. It's fair to say that loved ones often have doubts, mainly due to concerns about the safety and long-term impacts of surgery. However, with a better understanding of what obesity is, how it develops and how it can be treated both effectively and safely, many of these doubts can usually be dispelled.

Finally, whilst this information is primarily aimed at those seeking weight loss support, there will be health professionals who are keen to gain a better understanding of obesity and its treatments, who can gain valuable insights as well.

Contents

Author Profile: Mr Bilal Alkhaffaf MBChB, PhD, FRCS

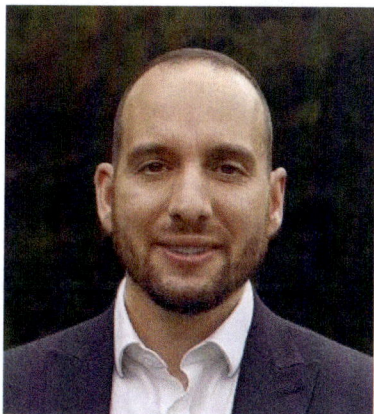

Bilal Alkhaffaf is a consultant surgeon with over twenty years of surgical experience, more than ten of which have been as a consultant. Born in Birmingham, he grew up in the North of England and attended the University of Manchester from which he graduated in 2003. Bilal specialises in the treatment of conditions affecting the upper gastrointestinal tract and offers the entire range of surgical and non-surgical weight loss procedures including the sleeve gastrectomy, gastric bypass (both full and mini bypasses), gastric balloon, gastric band, and revisional surgery.

Mr Alkhaffaf was appointed as a consultant surgeon in 2013 and his NHS practice is at Salford Royal Hospital (Northern Care Alliance Foundation Trust, Manchester) – the UK's largest specialist upper gastrointestinal centre. He is an expert in advanced minimally invasive (keyhole) surgery and trained at some of the most established upper gastrointestinal centres in the country. Bilal has further developed his expertise by visiting international centres of excellence in the United States, South Korea and The Netherlands as well as several leading institutions in the United Kingdom.

Bilal is active in the field of teaching and research and holds the position of Honorary Senior Lecturer at the University of Manchester. His international research activity has resulted in an award of a prestigious 'NIHR Doctoral Research Fellowship'. Mr Alkhaffaf has a particular interest in the way surgical outcomes (results from surgery) are reported, and in 2020 was awarded a PhD in this field. In 2016 he developed an international Fellowship programme for surgeons from abroad wishing to undertake further training in the field of upper gastrointestinal surgery.

Reflections from our patients

This guide focuses on the most important topics that should be considered in relation to weight loss treatments. However, the perspective of those who have undergone these life-changing procedures offers a unique insight which is also important to hear. Below are the reflections of just a few of the many patients we have treated over the years which will be referred to throughout this guidebook.

"It is the best decision I ever made."

"Surgery has changed my life. I've been able to get my confidence back; I've got the confidence to be myself again."

"I'm a lot happier and healthier after weight loss surgery."

"I feel physically and mentally so much better; I am active, back to playing sports. I love experiencing new adventures in life I never thought possible when I was overweight. My confidence has grown no end and continues to do so."

"Weight loss surgery has changed my life; I am fitter, going to work is easier, my health problems are disappearing. It has been a fantastic experience."

"I have got my quality of life back. Before my gastric sleeve I was depressed, unhappy, struggling with mobility and health issues, constantly poorly with breathing difficulties and other ailments. And now I am 6 stone lighter and healthier, and happy. I wish I had done it years ago."

"I am a much fitter and happier person now."

"The surgery has worked and I'm now a healthier, happier person."

"Weight loss surgery has completely changed my life."

"The surgery has changed my life for the better, and I will always be grateful."

"I am now living the healthy and active life that I have struggled to find for many decades."

Introduction

Each year my team speak to hundreds of men and women who have struggled with their weight and are desperate for help. Most have suffered years, decades and even a lifetime of feelings of failure, shame, self-loathing, and low self-esteem. Many are trapped in a never-ending cycle of dieting, weight loss, and weight regain without any clear way out.

Often people have seen significant effects on their physical and mental health, quality of life and overall wellbeing. Perhaps they need urgent treatments such as cancer surgery, joint replacement surgery, or even fertility treatments which they can't access until they've lost weight.

Some will have felt the social impacts of their weight; been treated differently by others, perhaps watched opportunities at work pass them by. Most parents tell me how they are unable to participate in family life as they want to, watching their children grow up without the parent they need. Many people are often afraid of what the future may bring, especially if they have parents, siblings or friends who have had similar challenges and suffered some of the devastating consequences of weight-related conditions such as diabetes, heart disease or strokes.

In my experience, everyone I speak to has exhausted every diet under the sun, subscribed to supervised weight loss programmes, taken up exercise, hired personal trainers, tried therapy, medications and sometimes even hypnosis. Despite these approaches, they have not seen the results for which they are desperate.

If these examples resonate with you, then I want to tell you that there is hope, and that the reason for your struggle is a lot more complex than you think. Importantly, there are safe, well-established, and powerful treatments which result in unparalleled, sustained weight loss, and significant improvements to - and in many cases complete reversal of - weight-related medical conditions. Whilst these treatments are not a magic solution that will fix everything for you, together with other changes, they can provide you with a powerful tool to use against your struggle with obesity.

So, if you or a loved one are considering medical treatments and surgery to help manage your weight more effectively, join us as we explore the topic of obesity and describe the powerful treatments which have helped millions of people around the world take back control.

Chapter 1: Obesity is not a 'choice'

What is covered in this chapter?

- What obesity is and how it develops.
- The importance of treating obesity.
- Common conditions linked to obesity.

Introduction

In this chapter, we will explore the topic of obesity, define what it is, understand how it develops, and begin to introduce some of the principles on which medical treatments are based. Obesity is probably one of the most misunderstood topics within healthcare. Many people – including a large proportion of medical professionals – incorrectly believe it develops because of laziness, a lack of willpower, or simply overeating. As a result, there is lots of prejudice and stigma aimed at those living with obesity both within healthcare and wider society. It is important therefore, to correctly understand obesity as a condition (which affects millions of people around the world) so that we can break down these myths and begin to put together effective strategies to manage it.

What is obesity?

Obesity can be defined as the excessive accumulation of fat which, importantly, poses a risk to health. It is a chronic, progressing, complex and relapsing condition, often affecting people for long periods of their life. In other words, it doesn't happen overnight, many factors contribute to it, and even if you lose a significant amount of weight, it is common to regain weight.

From a medical perspective, we often use the term 'body mass index' or BMI to define obesity. BMI considers a person's weight in relation to their height, with a 'normal' BMI being between 18.5 and 25 kg/m². A person is defined as having obesity if their BMI is greater than 30 kg/m². It is at this point that the risk of weight-related medical conditions increases significantly.

Accuracy of 'BMI' in defining obesity

BMI is often used by health professionals because it is easy to calculate, requires no specialist equipment, and is a reasonable guide with respect to health risks; the higher your BMI, the greater the risk is to your health.

However, BMI is not a perfect instrument. The current definition of obesity is based on historical records which don't consider key individual factors such as a person's genetics and biology, ethnicity, bone density or muscle mass. For example, whilst we know that Caucasian populations have a significantly higher risk of developing type 2 diabetes at a BMI of 30 kg/m^2, the same increased risk occurs at much lower BMIs for people of South Asian (BMI 24 kg/m^2) or Middle Eastern origin (BMI 26.5 kg/m^2).

In addition, BMI does not consider a person's pattern of fat distribution. There is extensive research which suggests that people who carry most of their weight above their waist and around their internal organs (often described as 'apple' shaped) have a much greater risk of developing conditions such as heart disease and diabetes, compared to people who carry their weight below their waist, around their bottoms and legs (often described as 'pear' shaped).

More recently, there has been a move to use other simple approaches to measure health risk. One alternative includes the waist to height (WHtR) ratio, which may be a more useful tool in people with a BMI of less than 35 kg/m^2. Using centimetres or inches for both numbers, a ratio of less than 0.5 indicates a 'healthy' range. 0.5 to 0.6 suggests a higher risk of obesity related conditions whilst 0.61 and above suggest a high risk. So, whilst BMI is an important guide, it is by no means perfect, and other factors should be considered when assessing obesity and risks to health.

The importance of treating obesity

Obesity is strongly linked to more than two hundred medical conditions, many of which result in a poorer quality of life, negative impacts on physical and mental health, and a shorter life expectancy. Some of these include diabetes, heart disease, stroke, high blood pressure, liver disease, cancer, and infertility. With respect to mental health, depression and anxiety, low self-esteem, poor body image and self-harm or suicidal ideation can also be a significant feature for many.

We also know that carrying excess fat, in and of itself, causes serious effects on mobility and joint health (particularly the back, hips and knees), but it also affects breathing and can lead to serious conditions including obstructive sleep apnoea.

Impacts of obesity can also be felt from a social perspective. People living with obesity are more likely to be discriminated against and stigmatised, and less likely to be offered employment opportunities. There are also wider implications on society such as the financial cost of healthcare linked to weight-related medical conditions. The current estimated cost to the UK's National Health Service (NHS) is over £6.5billion each year. However, the broader cost to society, when we begin to consider time off work for illness and the effect on social care for example, is estimated to take us closer to £30b a year.

Two-thirds of adults in the UK live with overweight or obesity, whilst 1 in 4 children are affected. This means that obesity is not a matter that can be brushed under the carpet. We also know that obesity doesn't affect everyone equally; it seems to be more common in people from deprived areas, older age groups, some black and ethnic minority groups, and people with disabilities.

Obesity is therefore an extremely serious condition affecting individuals and wider society which requires urgent attention so that it can be treated in those who have developed it and prevented in the wider population.

Common conditions linked to obesity

Let's take a closer look at some of the commonest weight-related medical problems that we see in people living with obesity and understand their impact on health. Whilst most of these conditions can require treatments such as medications to control, the good news is that many can be significantly improved or completely reversed through weight loss, improved nutrition and increasing levels of physical activity.

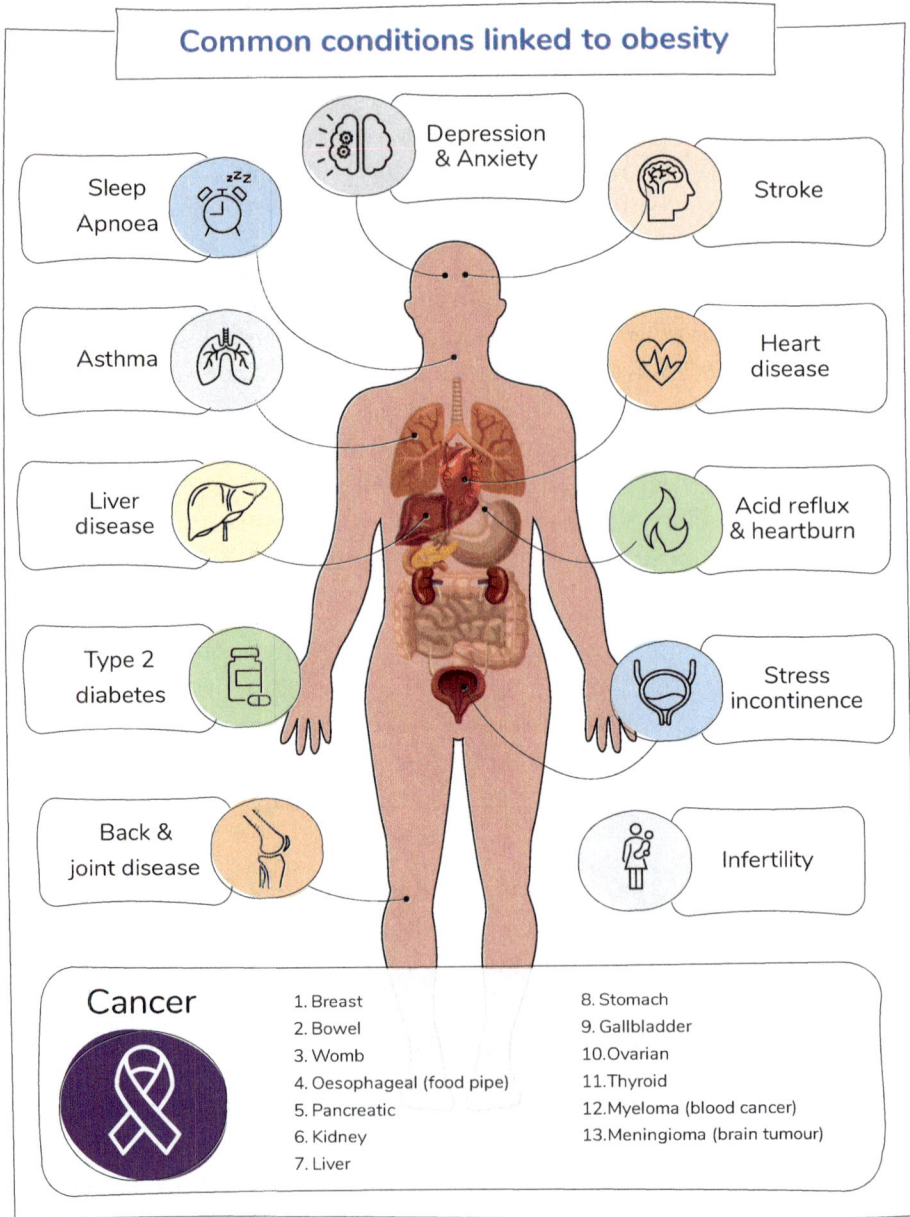

Common conditions linked to obesity

Depression & Anxiety

Sleep Apnoea

Stroke

Asthma

Heart disease

Liver disease

Acid reflux & heartburn

Type 2 diabetes

Stress incontinence

Back & joint disease

Infertility

Cancer

1. Breast
2. Bowel
3. Womb
4. Oesophageal (food pipe)
5. Pancreatic
6. Kidney
7. Liver
8. Stomach
9. Gallbladder
10. Ovarian
11. Thyroid
12. Myeloma (blood cancer)
13. Meningioma (brain tumour)

Type 2 diabetes

Type 2 diabetes is a chronic condition that affects how your body processes carbohydrates (including starches and sugar). When you eat, your body turns food into glucose, which is a form of sugar that provides energy for your cells. Insulin, a hormone produced by your pancreas, helps your cells absorb and use glucose. However, in type 2 diabetes, either your body doesn't produce enough insulin, or your cells become resistant to its effects. This leads to a buildup of sugar in your blood, which can be harmful over time.

Elevated blood sugar levels can damage blood vessels and nerves, leading to a range of serious complications. Uncontrolled type 2 diabetes increases the risk of heart diseases, strokes, kidney problems, vision issues, and nerve damage, particularly in your feet and hands.

High blood pressure

High blood pressure, also known as hypertension, is a common condition where the force of your blood against the walls of your arteries is consistently too high. Arteries are the blood vessels that carry blood from your heart to the rest of your body. When your blood pressure is consistently high, it can strain your arteries and organs, potentially leading to serious health problems.

High blood pressure places extra stress on your heart, making it work harder to pump blood. Over time, this increased workload can weaken the heart and increase the risk of heart diseases, heart attacks, and heart failure. Additionally, the continuous strain on your arteries can lead to their damage, increasing the chances of strokes, kidney problems, and other complications.

High cholesterol

Cholesterol is a waxy substance found in your blood which your body needs to build healthy cells. However, having high levels of cholesterol, particularly low-density lipoprotein (LDL) cholesterol, often referred to as "bad" cholesterol, can lead to a buildup of plaque in your arteries. This plaque buildup can narrow your arteries and restrict blood flow, potentially leading to serious health issues.

When there's too much LDL cholesterol in your blood, it can gradually accumulate on the walls of your arteries, making them less flexible and causing a condition known as atherosclerosis. This condition can reduce blood flow and oxygen supply to vital organs, increasing the risk of heart diseases, heart attacks, strokes, and other cardiovascular problems.

Heart disease

Heart disease, also known as cardiovascular disease, encompasses a range of conditions that affect the heart and blood vessels. It includes conditions like coronary artery disease, heart failure, arrhythmias (irregular heartbeat), and more. Heart disease often develops over time due to factors such as high blood pressure, high cholesterol, smoking, diabetes, and an unhealthy lifestyle including poor diet and inadequate levels of physical activity.

Heart disease is a leading cause of death worldwide. It can lead to heart attacks, strokes, heart failure, and other serious complications. The narrowing or blocking of blood vessels due to a buildup of plaque can reduce blood flow to vital organs, including the heart and brain, increasing the risk of life-threatening events.

Fatty liver disease

Non-Alcoholic Fatty Liver Disease (NAFLD) is a condition in which fat accumulates in the liver cells of individuals who don't particularly consume excessive amounts of alcohol. It's closely linked to factors such as obesity, insulin resistance, type 2 diabetes, and metabolic syndrome (a group of conditions occurring together including type 2 diabetes, high cholesterol and high blood pressure). NAFLD is a spectrum, ranging from simple fatty liver (steatosis) to more severe forms involving inflammation and scarring.

This damage can impair liver function over time and increase the risk of complications such as cirrhosis and liver cancer. The condition often develops silently without noticeable symptoms in its early stages.

Sleep apnoea

Obstructive sleep apnoea or OSA is a common sleep disorder characterized by pauses in breathing or shallow breaths during sleep. It occurs when the muscles in the back of the throat fail to keep the airway open during sleep, despite the effort to breathe. As a result, the airway becomes partially or completely blocked. These pauses can last for a few seconds to several minutes and can occur multiple times throughout the night, disrupting the quality of sleep and leading to symptoms such as loud snoring, gasping, or choking during sleep, and excessive daytime sleepiness.

OSA can affect individuals of any age, but it is more common in those who are overweight, have a family history of the condition, or have certain anatomical features that narrow the airway, such as a large tongue, tonsils, or a small jaw. Other risk factors include smoking, alcohol use, and certain medications.

OSA can lead to poor sleep quality, daytime sleepiness, and reduced overall well-being. The frequent drops in blood oxygen levels that occur during apnoea's (breathing pauses) can strain the cardiovascular system, increasing the risk of high blood pressure, heart diseases, strokes, and other health issues.

Cancer

Obesity is a well-established risk factor for at least 13 types of cancer. These include breast, bowel (colorectal), womb, oesophageal (food pipe), pancreatic, kidney, liver, stomach, gallbladder, ovarian, thyroid, myeloma (blood cancer), and meningioma (brain tumour). The relationship between obesity and cancer is complex, but there are several mechanisms through which obesity can increase the risk of developing cancer:

- Inflammation: Obesity is associated with chronic low-grade inflammation in the body. This inflammation can promote the growth of cancer cells and increase the risk of cancer development.
- Hormone Levels: Obesity can lead to hormonal changes, such as increased levels of insulin and oestrogen. Elevated insulin levels may promote the growth of cancer cells, while higher oestrogen levels are linked to breast and endometrial cancers.
- Insulin Resistance: Obesity is a major driver of insulin resistance, a condition in which the body's cells do not respond effectively to insulin. Insulin resistance is associated with an increased risk of several cancers, including colorectal cancer.
- Fat Tissue: Fat tissue, especially abdominal fat, produces hormones and other substances that can affect cell growth and promote cancer development.
- Immune System Function: Obesity can impair the function of the immune system, making it less effective at detecting and eliminating cancer cells.
- Changes in Gut environment: Obesity has been linked to changes in the composition of the gut microbiota (bacteria and other

organisms), which can affect inflammation and metabolism and potentially influence cancer risk.

It's important to note that while obesity is a significant risk factor, not all people living with obesity will develop cancer, and not all cancer cases are related to obesity. However, maintaining a healthy weight can significantly reduce the risk of developing. Additionally, regular cancer screenings and early detection are crucial for improving outcomes in cancer prevention and treatment.

Infertility

Obesity can significantly impact fertility in both men and women. Excess body weight can disrupt hormonal balance, affecting ovulation in women and sperm production in men. It's also linked to conditions such as polycystic ovary syndrome (PCOS) and insulin resistance, which further contribute to fertility challenges.

Obesity-related infertility can delay or prevent conception, leading to emotional stress and frustration for couples trying to conceive. In women, irregular menstrual cycles and ovulation difficulties can reduce the chances of getting pregnant. In men, obesity can lead to lower testosterone levels and reduced sperm quality.

Musculo-skeletal problems

Obesity can significantly impact the health of your back and joints. The excess weight places added stress on these areas, leading to increased wear and tear on the joints, particularly weight-bearing ones like the knees and hips. This can contribute to conditions such as osteoarthritis.

Obesity-related back and joint problems can result in chronic pain, reduced mobility, and a decreased quality of life. The pressure on joints can accelerate the breakdown of cartilage, leading to inflammation, pain, and decreased joint function. Chronic back pain can be debilitating and affect everyday activities.

Acid reflux & GORD

Gastro-oesophageal reflux disease (commonly known as GORD in the UK or GERD in the USA) is a chronic condition where stomach acid flows back into the oesophagus, causing symptoms like heartburn and regurgitation.

Obesity is a significant risk factor for GORD, as excess abdominal fat can increase pressure on the stomach, promoting the upward movement of acid into the oesophagus. This same process can result in part of the stomach protruding through the diaphragm, resulting in a condition called hiatus hernia.

Obesity-related GORD can lead to persistent discomfort, impacting daily life. The frequent exposure of the oesophagus to stomach acid can result in inflammation and damage to the lining, increasing the risk of complications such as oesophageal ulcers, strictures, and Barrett's oesophagus, a precancerous condition.

Stress urinary incontinence

Stress urinary incontinence (SUI) is a common condition where there is involuntary leakage of urine during activities that increase intra-abdominal pressure, such as sneezing, laughing, or lifting. Obesity can contribute to SUI by placing extra pressure on the pelvic floor muscles and weakening the supportive tissues that control bladder function.

Obesity-related stress incontinence can have a significant impact on daily life and emotional well-being. The loss of bladder control can lead to embarrassment, social isolation, and reduced quality of life. Additionally, untreated SUI may lead to skin irritation and urinary tract infections.

Impacts on mental health

Obesity can have significant effects on mental health. The relationship between obesity and mental well-being is complex and often bidirectional. So, while obesity can contribute to mental health issues, mental health challenges can also influence obesity. For example, obesity can reduce your ability to exercise, which in turn contributes to feelings of self-loathing, consequently resulting in behaviours that contribute to weight gain.

Obesity-related stigma, body image concerns, and societal pressures can lead to negative feelings about oneself, causing or exacerbating conditions like depression, anxiety, and low self-esteem. Additionally, obesity-related health problems and limitations can lead to reduced quality of life, increased psychological distress, depression, and anxiety. In

There are of course many more conditions (well over 200 as we have discussed) that are linked to obesity. The key message, however, is that these and many others can be reversed or significantly improved through weight loss and other lifestyle modifications.

How does obesity develop?

To understand how obesity develops, we must first appreciate some basic concepts with respect to how energy is used and stored by the body. The human body needs energy (which it gets from food and drink) to perform tasks such as basic metabolism, digestion of food, normal daily activities, and of course, exercise.

Up to a certain point, we know that if more energy than we need is consumed, the body stores it as fat. The opposite is also true that, if we consume less energy than we need, the body burns stored energy in fat, and weight loss occurs.

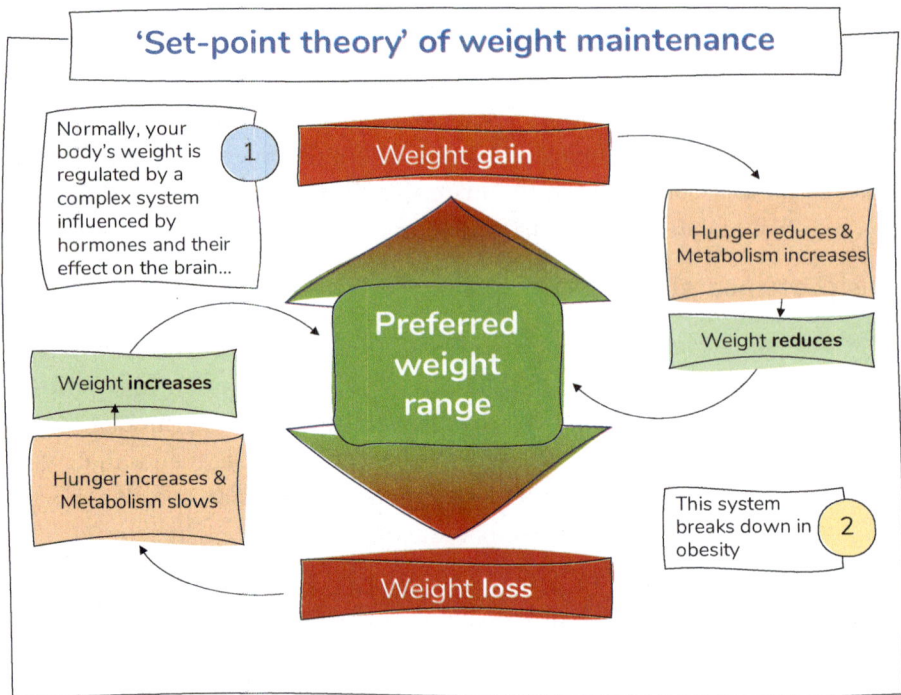

'Set-point theory' of weight maintenance

Normally, your body's weight is regulated by a complex system influenced by hormones and their effect on the brain...

1

Weight **gain**

Hunger reduces & Metabolism increases

Weight **reduces**

Preferred weight range

Weight **increases**

Hunger increases & Metabolism slows

This system breaks down in obesity

2

Weight **loss**

However, research suggests that in normal circumstances, the body can *control* the amount of fat it stores through a complex system influenced by hormones and their effect on the brain. This system works to maintain a 'set

16

point' or a preferred 'weight range' and will fight off attempts to change this significantly. This survival mechanism mirrors many of the other systems that the body uses to keep us healthy and in balance. When we increase our fat stores, the body responds by reducing hunger levels and increasing metabolism, resulting in weight loss. The opposite is also true that when we lose weight, the body increases hunger levels and reduces metabolism, resulting in weight gain.

This system can be compared to a heating thermostat; when the temperature drops too low, the heating system switches on and when the temperature becomes too high, the heating switches off to maintain the correct temperature. If you consider that throughout human history (up until the last 50 years or so) that food was difficult to come by, you can begin to understand the importance of such a system to human survival.

You may ask then, if there is a protective mechanism against significant weight change, why does obesity occur? In short, research suggests that several factors combine to create a 'perfect storm' which results in dysfunction of this protective mechanism. In other words, the body's systems can only withstand a certain amount of stress and pressure before it breaks down. Over time, this pressure leads to the body working to maintain a higher and higher 'set point' weight range, making it more and more difficult to lose weight through lifestyle changes alone.

The greater your weight, the more challenging it is to return to a healthy weight for the reasons already described. Research suggests that more than 90% of people living with obesity are unable to achieve and sustain significant weight loss through lifestyle changes alone. This is not a defeatist attitude but is key to helping both healthcare professionals and the wider public understand that other treatments *combined* with lifestyle modifications are often required to effectively treat obesity and maintain weight loss in the long-term.

The causes of obesity

There is no single cause for obesity, and often when we explore the background of someone living with obesity, we find several contributing factors are present. These factors may be individual, some may occur within our environments, some may be modifiable (in other words changeable) and some may be more difficult to influence. No two people are the same, and often, obesity occurs because of all these factors to a greater or lesser extent.

Some of the examples that most commonly contribute to the development of obesity in people we treat include:

- Poor diet and nutrition
- Reduced levels of physical activity
- Different medical conditions and medications
- High levels of stress (both acute or chronic)
- The impact of biology and genetics
- and of course, we mustn't ignore wider social and economic influences.

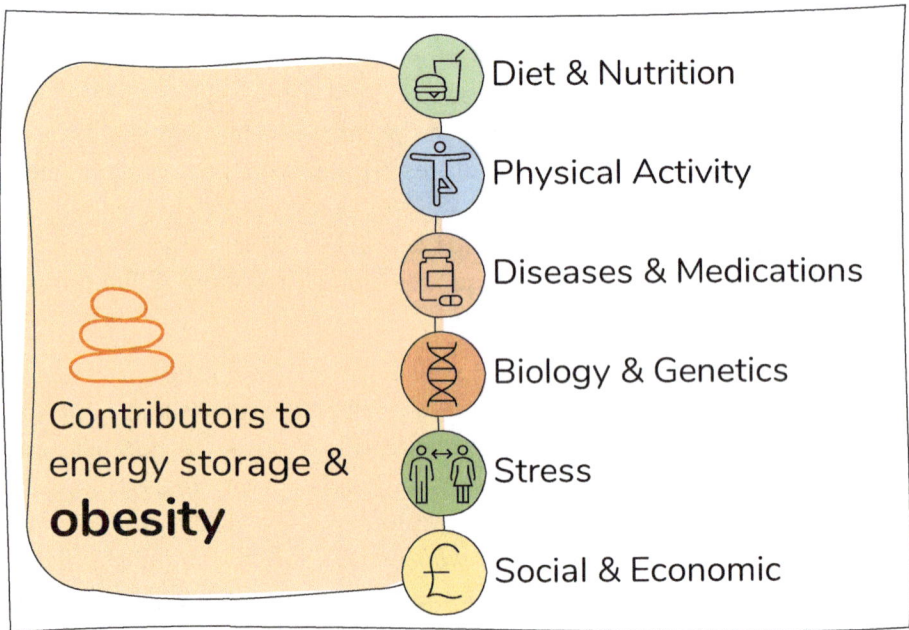

Contributors to energy storage & **obesity**

Diet & Nutrition

Physical Activity

Diseases & Medications

Biology & Genetics

Stress

Social & Economic

Diet and nutrition

There is well-established research which outlines how our eating behaviours result in weight gain. Not only do we need to consider the amount of food and drink we consume, but we should also pay close attention to the timing of meals as well as the type of food choices we make. Consuming highly processed foods, including those which contain refined sugars, additives, and preservatives, can cause us to feel hungrier compared to more balanced diets, and can also result in long-term changes to the gut environment and the microbes within it, which favour weight-gain.

We eat our emotions; our eating behaviours are *heavily* influenced by our feelings and emotions. We eat when we are hungry, but we also eat when we're happy, sad, stressed, bored and tired. Often our choices of foods in these circumstances are not good ones. It is also worth noting that during periods of emotional eating, portion sizes at mealtimes may be controlled, but binge eating and cravings can occur at other times.

Extreme calorie restriction diets can also have a negative effect on our weight in the longer term. Suddenly and significantly reducing your calorie intake results in a slowing down of metabolism, increased levels of hunger and food seeking behaviours, and ironically can result in you eventually putting on more weight than you started off with.

Reduced levels of physical activity

Over the last few decades, we have seen significant reductions in levels of physical activity and amount of time people spend moving. More of us drive to work where we sit at a desk, drive back home and then possibly relax in front of the TV. We spend more time on screens than we have ever done before, and this of course leads to us storing more of the energy that we consume.

The World Health Organisation (WHO) currently recommends that adults should undertake at least 150-300 minutes moderate intensity or 75-150 minutes of vigorous intensity activity each week. However, reductions in levels of physical activity may not always be a choice. Lots of people I speak to suffer from joint disease or pain which results in limited mobility. Some people may also have been involved in accidents or suffered physical trauma, and that certainly needs to be considered. Of course, most people will find mobility more and more challenging as their weight increases, further feeding into a vicious negative cycle of self-loathing, which in turn can limit their willingness to participate in physical activity in public.

Medical conditions & medications

Certain medical conditions such as an under-active thyroid, polycystic ovary syndrome (PCOS) and Cushing's disease can affect the body's hormonal balances and are directly linked to weight gain and the inability to lose weight.

Common mental health disorders such as depression and anxiety are also linked to obesity, as is neurodiversity including autism spectrum disorder (ASD) and attention deficit hyperactivity disorder (ADHD). These can lead to disordered eating behaviours that favour poorer nutritional choices and ultimately result in weight gain.

But many medications, which are often ironically used to treat weight-related medical conditions, are also directly linked to weight-gain. Examples include:

- Insulin and other anti-diabetic medications
- Certain types of blood pressure medications
- Some painkillers
- Steroids
- Specific anti-depressants
- Some anti-psychotics and anti-epileptics
- Oral Contraceptives
- And antihistamines

These can all contribute to weight gain and obesity through a variety of different mechanisms. In addition, these medications also have lots of other side effects which can impact negatively on quality of life.

Stress

We know that stress, whether due to interpersonal conflict in the home or at work for example, results in high levels of the circulating steroid hormone cortisol which can contribute to weight-gain, and stress of course influences our eating behaviours. This can lead to fat being deposited particularly around the organs (known as visceral fat) which is more likely to increase the risk of developing serious conditions such as diabetes and heart disease.

Biology and genetics

Our genetic make-up heavily affects our metabolism and the body's response to our behaviours and environment. We all know people who despite not being particularly active, can eat and drink what they want and not put on any weight, whilst *your* response to the same diet may be to put on significant amounts of weight. Our weight is influenced by genetics to such a degree, that the best predictor of how much weight someone can lose after weight loss surgery is how well a first-degree relative has done following their operation.

Lots of other biological factors are strongly linked to obesity including increasing age, the menopause, pregnancy, and disordered sleep.

Social & economic factors

We should also acknowledge the wider factors that heavily influence behaviour. We live in a society which is heavily influenced by persuasive advertising that very few of us are immune to, whether that be with respect to consumer products such as the latest phones, skin care, cars, or of course food.

Extensive research shows that in general, junk food usually costs significantly less than healthier options. So, there are cost implications, particularly in lower income families and especially at a time where many people are under severe financial pressure.

But convenience also plays a significant role. A recent study showed that more deprived communities had a much greater concentration of fast-food outlets which undoubtedly influences the availability and choice of food types.

Summary

In summary, the development of obesity is often due to a complex combination of factors and not a 'choice' or down to a lack of 'willpower'. This understanding helps us realise that tackling obesity usually requires more than one approach to address several underlying factors, some of which may be down to the individual lifestyle and stressors, whilst others come from the environment around us.

Chapter 2: Weight loss treatments

What is covered in this chapter?

- How weight loss treatments work.
- Eligibility criteria for surgery.
- Safety and general risks.
- The team approach to weight loss.

Introduction

Before we take a closer look at the well-established treatments for weight loss, it is important to understand the principles on which they work, the additional benefits that can be achieved over and above weight loss, and who is eligible for these types of treatments.

In this chapter we will also cover the important topic of safety, risks and complications and the steps that are taken to minimise these.

A brief history of weight loss surgery

The origins of weight loss surgery (also known as bariatric surgery) can be traced back to the 1950s when surgeons first attempted to treat obesity by removing parts of the small intestine. These early surgeries were often unsuccessful and associated with very high rates of complications.

In the 1960s and 1970s, advances in surgical techniques and anaesthesia led to the development of more effective bariatric procedures, including the gastric bypass and an outdated procedure called the vertical banded gastroplasty (VBG). These procedures remained invasive and still carried with them significant risk, but they offered hope to many individuals struggling with obesity.

In the 1980s and 1990s, laparoscopic techniques (keyhole surgery using very small incisions) began to make their way into the field of bariatric surgery, reducing complication rates and recovery time for patients. The introduction of the laparoscopic adjustable gastric band and the sleeve gastrectomy in the 1990s further expanded the options available to patients.

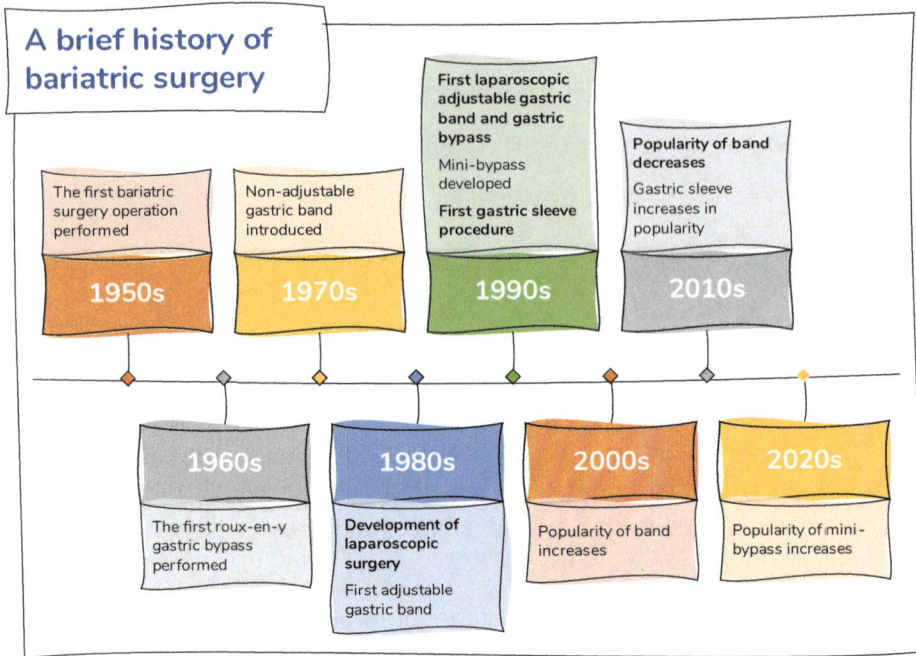

A brief history of bariatric surgery

First laparoscopic adjustable gastric band and gastric bypass

Mini-bypass developed

First gastric sleeve procedure

Popularity of band decreases

Gastric sleeve increases in popularity

The first bariatric surgery operation performed

Non-adjustable gastric band introduced

1950s
1970s
1990s
2010s

1960s
1980s
2000s
2020s

The first roux-en-y gastric bypass performed

Development of laparoscopic surgery

First adjustable gastric band

Popularity of band increases

Popularity of mini-bypass increases

Since the turn of the 21st century, bariatric surgery has become increasingly common and far more refined, with new techniques and technologies being developed all the time. These include the mini gastric bypass and much newer endoscopic procedures such as the endoscopic sleeve gastroplasty (also known as the ESG).

Today, bariatric surgery is recognised as an effective treatment for obesity, with significant benefits for patient health and quality of life. While the risks associated with the surgery have been greatly reduced, it is still of course a major medical procedure that requires careful consideration and consultation with a team of qualified medical professionals. The small risks of complications are covered in detail later.

How weight loss treatments work

Bariatric surgery is a field which is greatly misunderstood even amongst medical health professionals. There is often a misconception by many that these types of procedures are a type of cosmetic surgery, however, this is simply untrue and a misinformed view. These treatments also improve, and in many cases, completely reverse weight-related medical conditions. In other words, these treatments are as much about **health gain as they are about weight loss**. And whilst weight loss without doubt improves self-confidence and how we perceive ourselves, this is usually not the only and certainly often not the primary focus of patients when I speak with them in clinic.

It is important to recognize that treatments such as surgery do not 'cure' obesity; as we have already discussed, obesity is a progressive, long-term, and relapsing condition. Having a clear understanding of this allows us to appreciate that controlling weight requires a combination of long-term commitment and sustainable, effective tools. Surgery and other treatments are not 'an easy way out' and certainly not a magic solution that do all the work for you. By and large, you get out of the process what you put into it, the difference being that the results are usually incomparable to any other approaches to weight loss that most people have seen previously. These procedures must be combined with a **lifelong commitment** to lifestyle changes such as improved nutrition, sufficient levels of physical activity, and any other underlying factors that may have contributed to weight gain, must be addressed. Additionally, psychological support before and after surgery may be useful in trying to address factors related to eating habits; these may not be completely addressed, but controlling these will help significantly. This highlights the importance of support from a comprehensive team of experienced healthcare professionals which includes doctors, nurses, dietitians, physiotherapists, pharmacists, and psychologists.

Most people I speak to are stuck in a cycle of endless yo-yo dieting without a light at the end of the tunnel. This inevitably impacts on their mental health, self-esteem and ultimately the motivation to adopt the necessary choices which only results in further weight gain. Of course, we have already established that obesity is not caused by a lack of willpower alone, but motivation *is* necessary to make a change. The powerful effects of surgery provide some respite from the psychological trauma of obesity and gives you

25

the brain space and focus to be able to put into effect the necessary changes for long-term success.

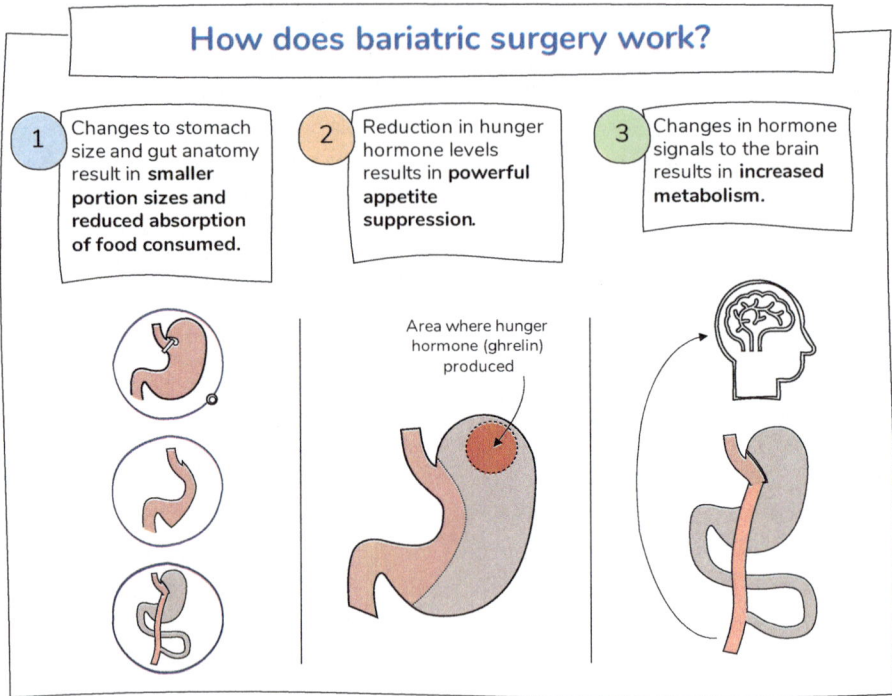

How does bariatric surgery work?

1. Changes to stomach size and gut anatomy result in **smaller portion sizes and reduced absorption of food consumed.**

2. Reduction in hunger hormone levels results in **powerful appetite suppression.**

3. Changes in hormone signals to the brain results in **increased metabolism.**

Area where hunger hormone (ghrelin) produced

It is said that insanity is defined as doing the same thing repeatedly and expecting a different result. As we will discuss, surgery (particularly the gastric bypass and gastric sleeve) gives us access to a different and far more powerful weight loss approach through changes in metabolism. Many people think that these procedures work simply by reducing the capacity of the stomach and therefore reducing the amount you can physically eat and drink. Whilst this is partly true, it does not describe the whole picture. If we compare two people on the same restrictive diet, one of whom has had bariatric surgery, the one who has undergone surgery will achieve significantly greater and sustained weight loss than the one on a restrictive diet alone. This is largely due to the physiological and hormonal changes that result in increased metabolism that are not seen in restrictive calorie diets. This manipulation of the body's metabolism is key to the success that most people see after surgery.

Finally, one size does not fit all. When I discuss the various available options, I will also make recommendations based on their unique set of circumstances, health-conditions, and personal goals. Surgery may not be appropriate for everyone. Sometimes it may even be necessary to postpone treatment until other health conditions such as diabetes, high blood pressure or sleep apnoea are better controlled. Making sure that any medical conditions are properly controlled ensures that the risks of surgery are as low as they can possibly be. Similarly, if there are psychological factors that that may impact negatively on your post-operative course, these will need to be addressed appropriately managed before surgery can proceed.

Ultimately, making sure that treatment options are tailored and safe will give you the best chance of controlling your weight and reversing weight-related medications conditions in the long-term.

Who should consider surgery and other treatments?

Guidelines and criteria

There are well-established national and international guidelines that help us decide who surgery is most appropriate for. This ensures that treatments can be delivered safely whilst offering the maximum possible benefits. We are also beginning to see a change in guidelines to support the safe use of these treatments in patients at a lower weight. It is therefore important to ask your team about the local criteria as this may be different from region to region.

Historically, if you have a body mass index of 40 kg/m² or more (with or without weight-related medical conditions) you would qualify for bariatric surgery. However, newer international guidelines suggest that this should be reduced to a BMI of 35 kg/m² with or without weight-related medical conditions.

If your BMI is 35 kg/m² or more with a condition that would benefit from weight loss, such as diabetes, high blood pressure, sleep apnoea or infertility for example, you would qualify for medical treatments such as surgery, however, newer guidelines suggest that this should be reduced to a BMI of 30 kg/m² or above. Some people may be offered surgery with a lower BMI depending on other factors such as their ethnic background or if they have been newly diagnosed with type 2 diabetes.

Other considerations

Whilst these criteria are important, they are not the only consideration. It is critical to understand a person's entire journey and their relationship with weight, diet, and other factors. When I talk to people considering surgery, most have struggled with their weight for many years and despite diets, personal trainers, and supervised weight loss programmes, they have been unable to lose a significant amount of weight or sustain long-term weight loss. Some may have tried medication or even had a previous procedure such as a gastric balloon or gastric band. There may also be a strong family history of obesity and related medical conditions, which may suggest a genetic predisposition to weight gain and developing certain life-threatening diseases.

All this information helps us piece together an understanding not just of your journey so far, but what the future may hold if medical weight loss treatments are not considered. So, whilst guidelines are vitally important to ensure safe practice by medical professionals, there is some flexibility that can be applied so long as there are strong grounds to do so.

Age restrictions

Another question I am often asked is whether there are age limits to bariatric surgery. The short answer is 'no'. The decision whether to offer surgery should be based on careful consideration of the risks and benefits regardless of age. There is a substantial body of evidence to support the safe use of surgery for people in their seventies as well as younger adults. There is also a strong argument that earlier treatments can help people avoid the years of psychological trauma and the physical impact that often accompanies obesity. Rather than being a 'last resort' to be used in later life, surgery should be seen as a powerful tool to be considered once reasonable attempts through lifestyle changes have been made. Certainly, the biggest regret I hear time and time again from my patients is **'I wish I had done it sooner'**.

Common reasons to consider weight loss surgery

Everyone's circumstances and impacts of obesity is unique to them. Therefore, the reasons for considering weight loss treatments will be usually different as well. Aside from weight loss of course, many people I speak to wish to improve their physical health by reversing or improving health conditions, or even reduce the risk of developing medical conditions before they occur. We can't ignore the fact that for many, being overweight affects self-confidence and contributes to conditions such as depression and anxiety, and for most people who are able to lose weight through surgery, we see significant improvements from this perspective. Many people wish to improve their mobility, particularly if obesity has resulted in joint or back pain.

All these factors often lead to serious impacts, and so improving overall quality of life and well-being is another leading reason for pursuing these treatments. Some patients are concerned about their life-expectancy, particularly if they have had parents or siblings who have suffered from years of chronic diseases, or even died suddenly from weight-related conditions such as heart disease and stroke. Many people wish to increase their energy levels perhaps to keep up with young children. Many women who have struggled with fertility will consider surgery either to improve their fertility or give themselves access to fertility treatments. Finally, many people may consider bariatric surgery to give themselves access to have other therapies such as cancer treatments and joint surgery which cannot be offered unless significant weight loss is achieved.

So, for people who meet the criteria and, with the support of a comprehensive team, commit to making lifestyle changes, and address other underlying factors, surgery can be a powerful tool in helping them achieve long-term and sustainable weight loss.

What are the benefits of bariatric surgery?

Bariatric surgery is the most powerful medical treatment available for obesity, resulting in long-term and sustainable weight loss. However, there are many other important benefits. Surgery extends life expectancy, results in improved quality of life and has major impacts on physical and mental health. Obesity is linked to over 200 medical conditions, some of which we have previously covered. Surgery results in significant improvements to, and often complete reversal of, many of these serious medical conditions including:

- Type 2 diabetes
- Heart disease

29

- High blood pressure
- High cholesterol
- Fatty liver disease
- Obstructive sleep apnoea
- Infertility
- Back and joint pain and
- Acid heartburn and reflux
- Urinary stress incontinence
- Anxiety, depression, and body image

And whilst for some patients some of these conditions never go away, at the very least, the number or dose of medications used can be significantly reduced. This is relevant as many of these medications can carry side effects. So, whilst most people consider bariatric surgery to reduce their weight, there are many other health benefits which can be achieved.

How successful is bariatric surgery?

Before we describe how successful surgery can be, we must first define what we mean by 'success'. Whilst for most, success means achieving a healthy weight, we have discussed how surgery also results in improved life expectancy, physical and mental health, and quality of life. So, success shouldn't just be measured by how much weight you lose.

With respect to weight loss, a person's ideal weight (which we define as a BMI of less than 25 kg/m^2) is not necessarily the best weight that can be achieved. There are lots of reasons for this, including the degree to which healthy lifestyle choices are adopted after surgery. However, there are other factors which can influence the amount of weight loss that can be achieved such as your age, genetics or biological factors, your starting weight, and a history of previous weight loss surgery and eating disorders.

- We know that younger patients tend to lose more weight than older patients.
- We also know that if you have a close (particularly first degree) relative who has lost a significant amount of weight with surgery, then there is a strong chance of you achieving good results as well.

- People who have a higher *starting* weight, may lose a larger total amount of weight compared to people who have less to lose, but may be less likely to achieve a BMI of 25 kg/m² or below.
- And finally, we know that results from revision surgery can be less predictable than first time surgery as we will discuss in greater detail later.

Another key consideration which impacts on the amount of weight loss is the type of procedure you undergo. We know that the gastric bypass and sleeve will result in more weight loss than the gastric band, which in turn results in greater weight loss than the gastric balloon and injectable medications.

Importantly, if you choose the right procedure and use it to help you make the necessary lifestyle changes, you will give yourself the best chance of losing a significant amount of weight, keeping it off in the long-term, and improving your general health.

Is bariatric surgery safe?

In short, weight loss surgery is **very safe and the risk of serious complications is extremely small**. Surgery is performed using a keyhole or laparoscopic approach (using very small incisions) which means that you can be discharged home with minimal pain and in most cases after just one night in hospital. Nonetheless, bariatric surgery is invasive, involves surgery on the stomach, and despite significant measures to reduce complications, these can never be completely eliminated. This highlights the importance of choosing your surgical team carefully and taking your time to understand the measures they have put in place to keep you safe.

Risks of serious complications related to bariatric surgery

Each of the different procedures has its own (low) rate of complications which we will cover later, at which point we will also discuss the signs to look out for during your recovery. However, let's begin by discussing what some of the most serious risks are.

The complication I am most often asked about is the **risk of dying** because of surgery. This is thankfully extremely rare and, in the UK, happens in less than 1 in 2000 cases. As a comparison, this is significantly lower than the risk from gallbladder or hip replacement surgery. The commonest causes for these rare events include serious infections, blood clots and heart attacks.

The **need for further treatment** (both in the short and long-term) to fix a problem which has occurred because of gastric bypass or sleeve gastrectomy surgery occurs in less than 5% of cases but can be much higher with the gastric band (particularly in the longer-term). Some of the reasons for these are discussed in further detail when we cover each procedure separately and under the topic of 'revision surgery'.

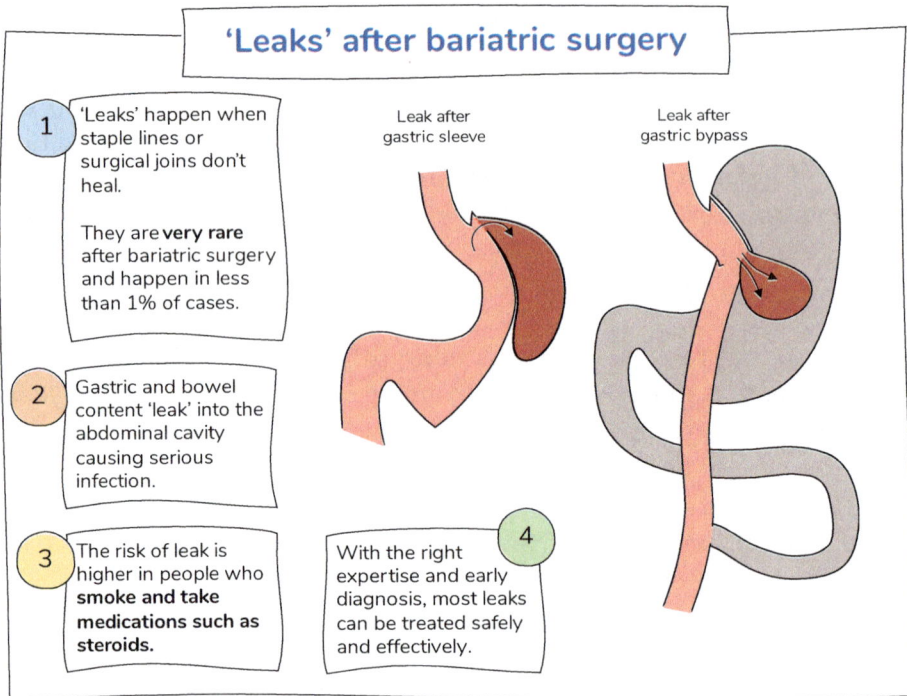

'Leaks' after bariatric surgery

1. 'Leaks' happen when staple lines or surgical joins don't heal.

   They are **very rare** after bariatric surgery and happen in less than 1% of cases.

2. Gastric and bowel content 'leak' into the abdominal cavity causing serious infection.

3. The risk of leak is higher in people who **smoke and take medications such as steroids.**

4. With the right expertise and early diagnosis, most leaks can be treated safely and effectively.

Leak after gastric sleeve

Leak after gastric bypass

A **leak** (sometimes called a perforation) occurs where the staple lines or surgical joins made during surgery do not heal properly. Consequently, stomach and bowel contents (which can include food, drink, and saliva) 'leaks' out of the gastrointestinal tract and into the abdominal cavity which can cause a serious and life-threatening infection if not treated. Leaks are very rare and occurs in less than 1% of cases, however the risk can be increased in smokers and in those who use medications that affect healing (such as steroids). If a leak occurs, further surgery and/or endoscopic treatment in a specialist bariatric centre is usually needed. With the right expertise and an early diagnosis, most leaks can be treated safely and effectively.

Bleeding is another rare complication and happens in less than 1% of cases. It can occur in any operation due to accidental injury to nearby blood vessels (for example near the spleen or in nearby fat), but bleeding can also happen from the gastrointestinal tract in procedures where the stomach or bowel is cut (such as the gastric sleeve or gastric bypass). Once diagnosed, bleeding sometimes needs further surgery or endoscopy to correct, alongside the use of blood transfusions other medications.

Finally, the risk of **blood clots** following bariatric surgery is also very low and occurs in less than 1% of cases. Blood clots can occur in the legs and arms (called deep vein thrombosis or 'DVT') and can be potentially life-threatening if they dislodge and travel to the lungs (called pulmonary embolism or 'PE'). Once diagnosed, treatment usually involves a course of blood thinning medications which might then be followed with longer-term medication (such as warfarin or newer drugs including apixaban) to reduce the risk of future clots. The small risk of blood clots can be increased in smokers, those with poor mobility (especially if you need a wheelchair or walking aids to mobilise), and if you have a past personal or family history of DVT. The topic of how the risk of DVT is reduced is covered in greater detail later.

Risks of anaesthesia and laparoscopic surgery

Another concern that some people have is the safety of having a general anaesthetic (being put to sleep) in the context of obesity. Again, the risks of general anaesthetic are extremely small and reduced further still by having an experienced anaesthetic team who undertake these procedures regularly. Other risks of laparoscopic or keyhole surgery include a small risk of bleeding (which we have already covered), unintended injury to nearby structures and organs, and infections (such as wound infections). The risk of these complications is small and occur in the region of less than 1% of procedures.

Minimising the risk of complications

Whilst the risks of surgery can never be eliminated entirely, there are several ways in which they can be significantly reduced. And on the rare occasion that problems arise, it is important to identify them early so that they can be addressed promptly, giving patients the best chance of a good outcome.

Ensuring that patients receive the **highest standards of care** is at the top of the list in terms of reducing risk. This is achieved through meticulous surgical technique based on the experience of undertaking hundreds of weight loss surgery procedures each year and using the highest quality equipment. In addition, it is important to make sure that the anaesthetic is undertaken by a team who are well versed in looking after patients with obesity. Finally, we can minimise risk by performing surgery in a hospital with access to specialist facilities such as a high dependency unit, and which offers round the clock access to emergency advice, which allows us to recognise and respond to problems early.

Working within **well-established and well-trained teams** means that patients are cared for by experts who are used to doing the same thing all the time. A lot of time and training is invested to ensure that team members in pre-operative assessment, theatre and on the wards understand the needs of patients having bariatric surgery. This means that mistakes are less likely to be made in the first place, but that team members are also actively on the lookout for problems. In addition, enhanced recovery programmes are commonly used to allow patients to be looked after in a standardised manner, again removing variation, and reducing the risk of complications.

There are several key **patient-related factors** which can affect the safety of surgery and ultimately how well recovery occurs. These should be identified during your initial consultation and the formal pre-operative assessment and will be covered later in greater detail. Some of the common issues that can increase the risk of complications include:

- The use of **nicotine** products: Using nicotine products such as cigarettes and vapes, which can affect healing and infection rates alongside certain medications such as steroids and biologics used in conditions such as rheumatoid arthritis.
- Use of certain **medications**: There may be a higher chance of bleeding if you take medications that thin the blood. On the other hand, if you take tablets containing oestrogen such as the combined oral contraceptive pill or hormone replacement therapy (HRT), there may be an increased chance of developing blood clots to the leg and lungs (also known as a deep vein thrombosis - DVT or pulmonary

embolism - PE). This risk may also be increased if you have a particular problem with mobility or a history of blood clots.

- The presence of previously undiagnosed **medical conditions**: If you have undiagnosed conditions such as obstructive sleep apnoea, this can affect recovery in the immediate post-operative period which is why you will be asked to answer questions which will help us understand the likelihood of whether or not you suffer from it.

- An **enlarged liver**: As we will cover later, the liver sits directly on top of the stomach and needs to be gently retracted out of the way to safely undertake bariatric surgery. A larger heavier liver may make it technically more challenging to undertake your surgery and in some rare cases, it may not be possible to undertake the procedure as planned.

As long as these factors are identified early on in the process and the appropriate steps taken to minimise their impact, there is no reason why they should result in a significantly higher risk of complications. However, this highlights the importance of a thorough approach to assessing patients before surgery.

How important is a team approach to weight loss?

In my opinion, the care and support you receive before and after surgery is as important as the procedure itself. Whilst surgery is a powerful tool in helping you lose weight, the long-term success of maintaining weight loss depends heavily on the correct lifestyle choices that you continue to make.

For example, most people will need help to reverse many years of learned behaviours with respect to diet, such as understanding what a balanced and varied meal looks like, what to eat, when to eat, and how often to eat. Others may have underlying psychological trauma which has resulted in them seeking comfort in food, and that of course will need to be addressed. Increasing levels of physical activity is vital; not just in terms of general levels of activity but also understanding how to build muscle mass which can contribute to an increased metabolism.

Whilst for most people, preparing for and recovering from surgery follows a relatively predictable pattern, there are some people who need additional support either from a medical, nutritional, or psychological perspective. Patients can often be worried about how pain and nausea symptoms are going to be managed after surgery as well. So having access to an experienced team of doctors, dietitians, specialist nurses, physiotherapists, pharmacists, and psychologists both in the lead up to and after surgery, is vitally important to recovering well from your procedure and achieving success in the long-term.

Team members you will meet along the way

A comprehensive approach to weight loss will involve the support of several key people in addition to a much wider network of team members who ensure that your care is delivered safely and effectively.

Surgeon

The surgeon is the doctor who performs your weight loss operation or procedure. Usually, they, alongside other members of the team, are responsible for your care in the lead up to, around the time of, and in the follow-up period after surgery.

It is important that your surgeon can offer a wide range of weight loss procedures and has the necessary experience to guide you through an informed decision-making process. Your surgeon should also have undergone the necessary training and undertake bariatric surgery regularly to be able to provide you with a safe procedure and a low risk of complications.

Medical physician

Medical doctors with an interest in weight management play an important role in the wider team but are also central to the provision of medical weight management treatments. It is common for medical physicians to oversee the administration of injectable weight loss medications as well as optimise weight-related medical issues such as diabetes ahead of surgery.

Bariatric nurse

The bariatric nurse is the key contact point for patients undergoing surgery and coordinates much of the patient education and post-operative care. They also play an important part in identifying and sorting problems. It is common for bariatric nurses to be involved in the pre-operative assessment process and depending on their training and expertise may also undertake some of the psychological screening assessments as well.

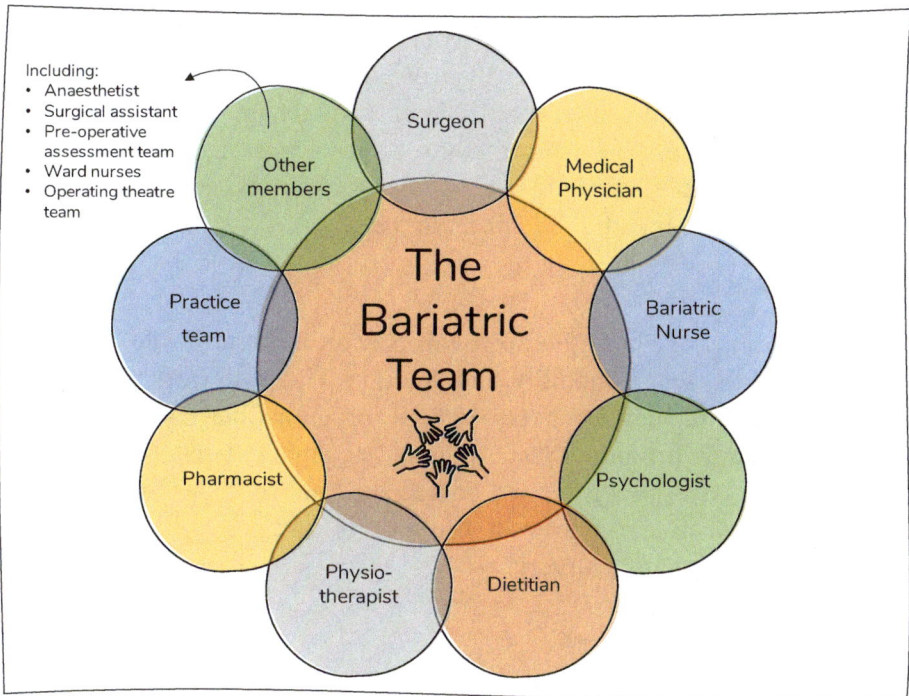

Including:
• Anaesthetist
• Surgical assistant
• Pre-operative assessment team
• Ward nurses
• Operating theatre team

Surgeon
Medical Physician
Other members
Practice team
The Bariatric Team
Bariatric Nurse
Pharmacist
Psychologist
Physio-therapist
Dietitian

Bariatric Psychologist

A psychologist with specialist training and expertise in the field of bariatric surgery may be involved in your initial pre-operative psychological assessment and will sometimes continue to offer support following surgery.

Psychologists play an important part in assessing a person's psychological preparedness for surgery, particularly in terms of exploring their patterns of eating and relationship with food, and understanding of what will be required after surgery. They will also highlight any potential areas of concern that may hamper recovery and progress, and which needs further exploration before surgery can proceed.

Bariatric Dietitian

A bariatric dietitian specialises in all thing's nutrition and food and will feature heavily in your post-operative follow-up. Most people will require a significant change to their diet and your dietitian will help you design a tailored eating plan for you. You will also require support and education as you progress through the different phases of recovery and develop the habits that will help sustain long-term control of your weight. Support and education from dietitians should begin before surgery and continue until you are discharged from the aftercare programme.

Physiotherapist

As you recover, a physiotherapist will play an important role in helping you regain your strength, mobility, and function. They will work closely with you to develop an individualized exercise program that can aid in your weight loss and promote your overall health and well-being. The physiotherapist will also give you advice on how to reduce the risks of complications, such as deep vein thrombosis and pneumonia which is especially important after surgery.

Pharmacist

Many patients who seek weight loss surgery take medications. After surgery, the doses may need to be altered or the way in which they are administered will need to be changed (for example, using liquid versions instead of tablets). Bariatric surgery can also affect the way in which certain drugs are absorbed, and there will also be new medications and supplements that will need to be taken after surgery. The bariatric pharmacist will coordinate this process for you and ensure that it is done safely, usually in liaison with the surgical and other specialist medical teams. The pharmacist is also pivotal in managing medication side effects as well as symptoms such as pain and nausea.

Practice Manager/administrative team:

The practice team or patient coordinators are usually the first port of call with respect to arranging the logistical aspects of your care, including booking an initial consultation with your surgeon. They will provide information regarding dates for surgery, paying for treatment, and will also arrange all follow-up consultations with your surgeon.

Other team members

There are many other people who you will meet during your journey, including the anaesthetist, surgical assistant, pre-operative assessment and ward nurses and members of the theatre team. All these team-members work closely together to make sure that your care is delivered safely and to the highest standards.

Choosing your team: Key considerations

In addition to choosing a weight loss procedure, you will also need to carefully consider the team who undertakes your treatment. Whilst bariatric surgery is safe, it is nonetheless invasive and requires the right expertise. There are currently lots of providers offering surgery, and not all offer the same levels of care or support. There has also been a significant rise in the number of people considering surgery abroad where procedures are often cheaper. Here we will discuss the main factors that you should consider when choosing where to have surgery.

Quality of Care

One of the most important considerations when having bariatric surgery is the quality of medical care you will receive. You should research the credentials, qualifications, and experience of the surgeon, as well as the reputation of the hospital or clinic where the surgery will be performed. Personal recommendations and online reviews can often give you an important insight. Make sure that the facility is accredited and has a good track record of positive patient outcomes. In the UK, all hospitals both in the NHS and the private sector must adhere to high standards of care and are regularly inspected by the independent Care Quality Commission.

The surgeons you speak to should be able to describe their experience and reliably tell you what their personal complication rates are. All UK surgeons must submit their outcomes to a national registry which is published publicly on a regular basis. If you are considering surgery abroad, you should consider that it *can* be difficult to know whether the facility and staff have the necessary qualifications and experience to perform the surgery safely.

Speak to more than one provider

Many people will contact more than one team, giving them an opportunity to consider the different levels of service on offer and a chance to speak to different surgeons. This is important as different surgeons may offer different perspectives with respect to treatment recommendations.

Aftercare

By now, it will be clear how critically important aftercare is to your journey and maintaining results in the longer term. Make sure you understand how long the aftercare package lasts and what is included, such as comprehensive pre-operative assessments, dietitian and psychology assessments, exercise recommendations, post-operative medication guidance and access to emergency care if this is needed. You should also be aware that routine aftercare is not usually provided by the NHS or private providers for patients undergoing surgery abroad.

Considerations Specific to Health Tourism

Undoubtedly there has been a rise in people considering surgery abroad, mainly because of limited access to publicly funded surgery and cut price offers alongside targeted advertising campaigns. This is a controversial topic which requires careful thought and consideration. In addition to the factors already described, there are more specific issues to consider.

If you are paying for surgery, the **financial cost** is naturally going to play a part in the decision-making process. It is therefore especially important to understand what the advertised costs include. There may be additional costs involved including travel expenses, health insurance, accommodation, and further medical care or follow-up visits that may be required. Be wary of cut-price deals. If it sounds too good to be true, it probably is. Cheap deals can indicate a lower standard of care in sub-standard facilities, the use of inferior quality, yet critically important equipment such as stapling devices, and of course little access to any meaningful aftercare.

Communication in healthcare is vitally important. If you are going to a country where the primary language is not your native language, you will need to consider the potential challenges of communicating with medical staff before, during, and after your treatment. Think carefully about how this may affect your care if you have any problems or complications after surgery.

Make sure that you are offered a translator or that the medical staff can communicate in a language you are comfortable with. There are also cultural considerations that you may not be aware of as a health tourist that can impact on your expectations in relation to care. Take the time to explore and understand these in advance of making decisions about surgery.

Different countries have different **regulations** and laws regarding bariatric surgery. Make sure that you research the legal requirements where you plan to have the surgery. You should also be aware of the regulatory bodies that govern weight loss treatments in case you need to make a complaint.

Depending on the type of bariatric procedure you have, you will need to take time to recover following this. If you work, there may be a period during which you will not be able to fulfil your duties (we will cover this in greater detail later). If you are having surgery abroad, you will need to factor in the **additional time needed for travel and recovery in a foreign country**. You will also need to be aware of additional risks of flying immediately after surgery, such as blood clots to the leg and lungs (DVT and PE) and ensure that measures to reduce these risks are offered. Finally make sure that the travel company you are with are willing to safely transfer you following invasive surgery, particularly if you have suffered a complication.

Summary

In summary, bariatric surgery is a safe, effective, and well-established approach to losing weight and improving health. Achieving the best results requires a combination of safely delivered treatment alongside changes to lifestyle and addressing other underlying factors. This is best done with the support of an experienced team of experts who provide this type of care on a regular basis. Finally, take your time to carefully research the team you wish to have your surgery with, as this will give you the confidence that the care you will receive will be of the highest quality.

Chapter 3: Introduction to weight loss procedures and non-surgical treatments

What is covered in this chapter?

- Choosing the right procedure for you.
- Non-surgical treatments.
- Novel treatments.

Introduction

Now that you have a better understanding of the principles on which weight loss treatments are based, let's delve further into the specific options available. Most people considering surgery and other treatments for weight loss will recognise that the internet provides unfettered access to information on this topic. Rather than being informative, this can lead to confusion and a lack of direction. In this chapter we will explore how you can begin to tease apart the wealth of information available, so you can make informed choices which will help you achieve long-term and sustained success.

There are now several well-established options available to support weight loss, including:

- Medical-weight management using medications and supervised weight loss
- The gastric balloon
- The adjustable gastric band
- The sleeve gastrectomy (also known as the gastric sleeve) and
- The full (roux-en-y or RNY) and 'mini' (one or single anastomosis) gastric bypasses

These treatments are tried and tested and importantly, we know about their benefits and downsides both in the short and long-term. In recent years we have also seen the emergence of more novel treatments such as injectable

43

medications, the endoscopic sleeve gastroplasty or ESG, and less invasive gastric balloons. In this section, we will introduce each of these procedures, focusing mainly on non-surgical options, describe how they work, discuss risks of complications specific to the procedure and cover reasons to consider them as a choice for weight loss.

Choosing the right weight loss procedure

The internet and social media have been instrumental in opening a door to the world of bariatric surgery. This has undoubtedly broken-down barriers to accessing information for many. You can now follow the lives of those who have undergone surgery and really understand the lived experience and what this may look like for you. Whilst this can be helpful in making decisions about whether to pursue weight loss surgery and which procedure may be best suited to you, the sheer amount of information available (and understanding how accurate and relevant it is to you) can also be overwhelming and confusing.

So how do you make sense of it all? My advice would be to try and adopt a balanced approach. It is important to undertake your own research on the topic initially, to understand whether bariatric surgery is something you wish to consider. However, it is also important that you speak to experienced healthcare professionals who work within the field and have a broader as well as a more nuanced understanding of how the different options may impact on your own set of circumstances.

It is vital to understand that there will never be a single choice available to you that offers only positives with no downsides. As we will discuss, every option (including the option of doing nothing) has a trade-off and this needs to be carefully considered. Sometimes, your set of circumstances may mean that you have to choose the least bad option to help achieve significant weight loss.

For example, our current understanding is that the sleeve gastrectomy can be linked to worsening heartburn symptoms, so if you already have significant acid reflux or heartburn, your consultation may focus on the benefits of the gastric bypass in that scenario. However, this needs to be balanced against the greater risk of longer-term nutritional problems and other issues related to the bypass, which is a more invasive procedure. This is particularly important in the younger patient group where extra thought needs to be placed with respect to the longer-term impacts and effects of surgery on health and well-being.

Our understanding of obesity has changed significantly over the last decade or so. We now recognise that obesity is a chronic and relapsing condition that requires long-term control. Often, patients may initially be drawn towards non-surgical options (such as a gastric balloon or injectable medications) or a gastric band because these are reversible and temporary treatments. However, many patients will change their mind once they understand that long-term tools are required to manage this long-term problem.

When considering which options to pursue, also keep in mind your own goals and aspirations. What is it that you want to achieve the most? For example, do you want to get your BMI down into the 20's? Or is it that your focus is more towards improving certain health conditions. If you want to maximise weight loss, it may be that you opt to go for a more invasive option such as a gastric sleeve or bypass, or even that you opt for a combination of multiple treatments (see below).

Another consideration is that whilst a bypass may be better at achieving slightly greater weight loss than the sleeve in the short-term, we also need to be mindful that there are currently very few effective strategies to address weight-regain after a bypass if it occurs. However, if weight regain occurs in the future in the context of a sleeve gastrectomy, there are further surgical options including a gastric bypass. These pragmatic considerations should be explored particularly in younger patients and may impact on decision-making.

Ultimately, these points and other considerations need to be discussed with your surgeon. Once again, this highlights the importance of ensuring that your bariatric team is experienced and can offer a range of options to suit your needs.

Choosing more than one approach

There are some circumstances where a combination of different treatments may be required as part of a strategy for weight loss. This most commonly occurs where a person's BMI is greater than $50kg/m^2$ and most certainly when the BMI is greater than $60kg/m^2$. As we have already discussed, the higher your starting weight, the lower the likelihood of achieving an ideal weight which takes you nearer a BMI in its 20's. In these scenarios, there is rarely a single procedure or treatment which will help you achieve all your desired weight loss. Whilst a BMI in its 20's isn't necessarily the only goal or even the definition of success for many people, for those looking to maximise weight loss, understanding this will help to keep your expectations realistic. We will discuss weight loss goals and the best ways to achieve them in greater detail later.

In situations where the starting weight is very high, I would usually advise a 'multi-modal' approach which may mean using a combination of injectable medications for a period, followed by a combination of surgical procedures. This may commonly begin with a sleeve gastrectomy followed by a gastric bypass 18 to 24 months later. If your starting weight is very high, make sure to speak to your surgeon to discuss realistic weight loss goals and approaches to maximise these.

The option of doing nothing

Most people who I speak already have a reasonable idea of what they want and how they want to achieve it. However, it is always important to consider the alternatives. The first alternative to medical treatments is, of course, to do nothing at all. This is the only option that completely eliminates the small risk from weight loss procedures. However, as we have covered, 90% of people living with obesity who use diet and exercise alone will not be able to lose a significant amount of weight or maintain that weight loss. Of course, not addressing your weight sufficiently may expose you to a higher risk of developing weight-related medical conditions in the future.

Important Anatomy

Before we explore different weight loss options, it is worthwhile briefly covering some basic human anatomy which may be affected by some of these treatments and procedures. Food is swallowed into the oesophagus (also known as the gullet or food pipe) before it then enters the stomach. The stomach is a muscular organ (approximately 15cm wide and 25cm long) which is found at the topmost portion of the abdominal cavity (behind lower end of the breastbone). It has many functions, such as the production of important hormones and chemicals (including acid) which are important for the digestion of food and the maintenance of gut health. One important hormone that is manipulated following bariatric surgery is ghrelin, which is responsible for the sensation of hunger.

Food and drink usually remain in the stomach for approximately 3-4 hours before it is released into the small intestines where important nutrients are absorbed. Similarly, the intestines (which are 4-6 metres in length) are critically important to the process of digestion and release important hormones, chemicals, and enzymes to aid this process. Like ghrelin, these are also altered by weight loss procedures (especially in the case of the sleeve gastrectomy and gastric bypass).

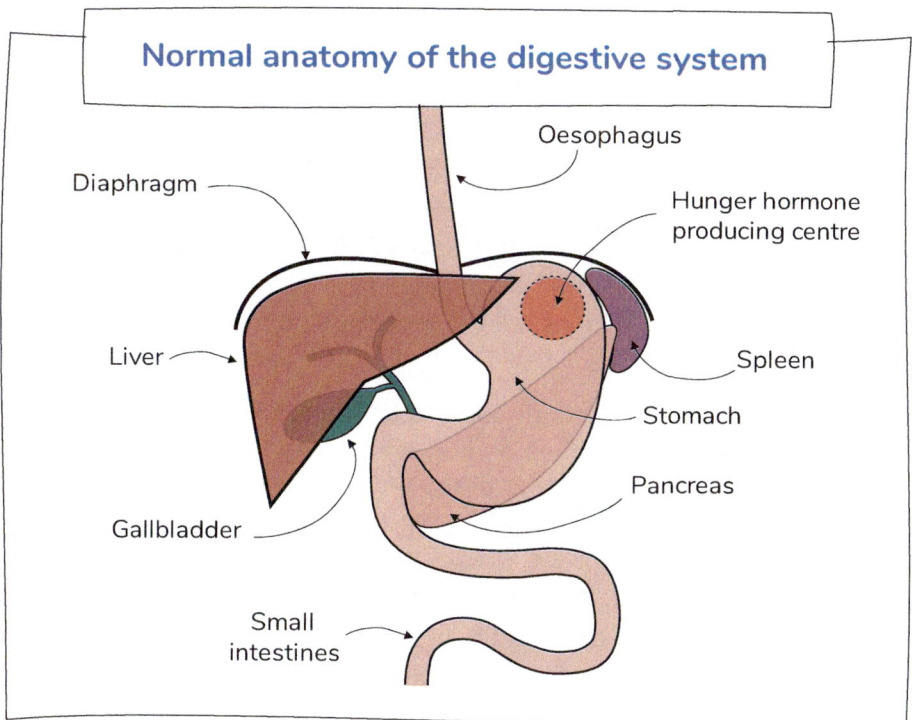

Normal anatomy of the digestive system

Oesophagus

Diaphragm

Hunger hormone producing centre

Liver

Spleen

Stomach

Pancreas

Gallbladder

Small intestines

The liver is a major organ which is found in the upper right area of the abdominal cavity that, amongst other roles, produces a chemical called bile. Bile is stored in the gallbladder and released to aid in the digestion of fats. The pancreas gland is found behind the stomach and in addition to producing digestive enzymes, is also responsible for controlling blood sugar levels by releasing a hormone called insulin. Next to the stomach, at the 'tail' of the pancreas gland is the spleen. The spleen is a major organ which plays an important role in immunity.

As we will discuss later, the function of the oesophagus, stomach, intestines, liver, gallbladder, and pancreas gland are all affected by both surgical and non-surgical treatments.

Medical Weight Management

What is it & how does it work?

Medical weight management involves supervised weight loss by a team of medical doctors, specialist bariatric nurses, dietitians and psychologists using a combination of approaches which may include weight loss medications such as injections called GLP-1 agonists (for example semaglutide and liraglutide). This is a rapidly expanding area which will likely see the development of many other medications to help manage weight. In combination with appropriate supervision (which cannot be underestimated), input from other specialists such as psychologists (to address eating behaviours), and changes in lifestyle choices, these injectable medications primarily work by suppressing appetite and increasing feelings of fulness.

GLP-1 agonists were first discovered in the 1980s when researchers identified GLP-1 as an important hormone in the regulation of glucose metabolism and insulin secretion. In the 1990s, it started to be used to help manage type 2 diabetes. More recently, GLP-1 agonists have been approved for use in obesity by the United States' Food and Drugs Agency (FDA) and the UK's National Institute for Health and Care Excellence (or NICE). This is a particularly exciting field within the field of obesity treatments, and we are likely going to see many more developments in this area over the coming decade.

As these medications are a relatively new introduction to treatments for the management of obesity, we don't have a lot of real-world data about their effectiveness – particularly in the long-term. On average, research studies have reported people losing between 8-15% of their body weight compared to those not receiving these medications.

Reasons to choose or avoid GLP-1 injectables

The main advantage of medical weight management is that it avoids the small risks of surgery, and weight loss may be sufficient to address some of the underlying weight-related medical conditions. For many people, it is often seen as an additional measure that can be taken before surgery is considered. We are also seeing the use of injectable medications either as a bridge to or in conjunction with more effective surgeries like the gastric sleeve or the bypass. Sometimes a person's weight may make the risk of surgery higher than we would want (for example if their BMI is greater than $60kg/m^2$), and so by reducing their weight beforehand, the technical challenge of undertaken surgery is reduced. Finally, these medications may be useful in patients who have already had surgery and have begun to regain weight.

If your body mass index is significantly higher than $35 kg/m^2$, it is unlikely that GLP-1 agonists alone will result in significant and sustained weight loss in the long-term. In addition, these medications are not a long-term option as they can only be prescribed for 2 years. Consequently, many people are seeing significant rates of weight regain when the medications are stopped. Finally, there is of course an ongoing cost implication for injectable medications, particularly if you pursue these treatments privately.

Potential Risks

As with any interventions, there can be downsides to these medications. As these medications have only recently been introduced to treat obesity, there is little long-term and 'real-world' information about side effects. This means that some side-effects may only be discovered many years down the line. Allergies or intolerances can occur which may manifest themselves as gastrointestinal symptoms such as diarrhoea and abdominal cramps, particularly as the dose is increased. This is especially the case as doses are increased when weight loss slows down. Rarely, GLP-1 agonists have been associated with inflammation of the pancreas gland or pancreatitis and there have been some concerns about the increased risk of developing thyroid cancer, although the evidence for this is mixed.

The gastric balloon

What it is and how it works

The gastric balloon is a temporary silicone device which is filled with fluid and sits in the stomach for up to 12 months. It works by restricting the amount of food and liquid you are able to consume and making you feel full.

The concept of using a balloon to aid weight loss dates back to the 1980s. The first fluid-filled silicone balloon was introduced in the 1990s. Over the years several modifications have been made to improve both its safety and effectiveness.

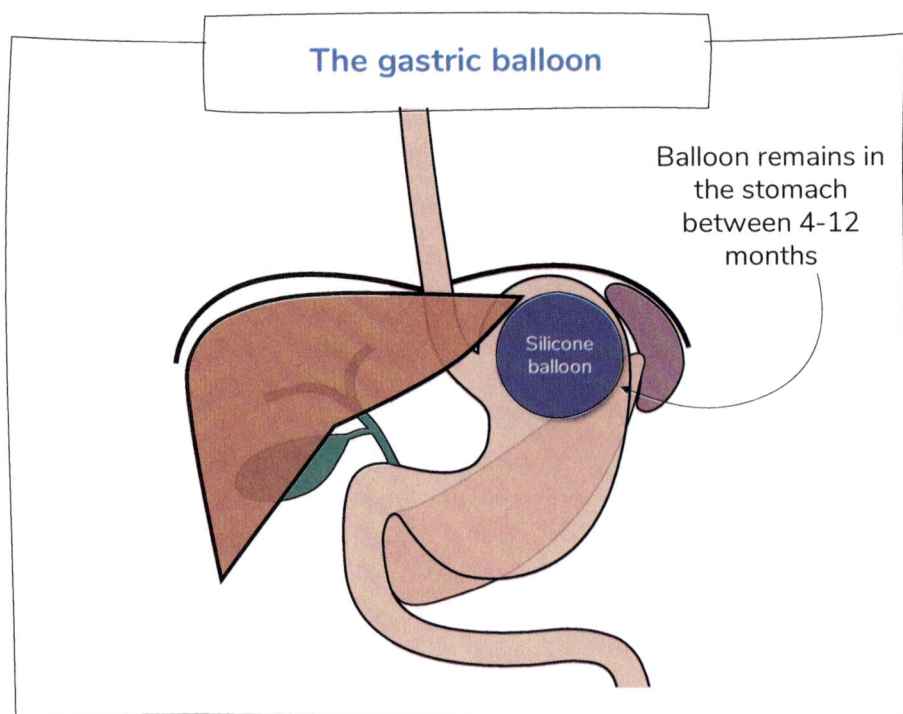

The gastric balloon

Balloon remains in the stomach between 4-12 months

Silicone balloon

How it is performed

Traditionally, the gastric balloon is inserted using a gastroscope (camera procedure sometime called an endoscope) which goes down the throat and into the stomach. Once in place, the balloon is filled with up to 500mls of fluid to keep the balloon inflated. The procedure is undertaken using sedation (which aims to significantly reduce your awareness without putting you completely to sleep) avoiding a general anaesthetic. The balloon is then removed either 6 or 12 months later at which point it is deflated and retrieved using a gastroscope.

More novel approaches which avoid the need for a gastroscope or sedation are also available. These balloons can be introduced in the outpatient clinic setting by swallowing a small balloon the size of a pill connected to a tube, which is then used to fill the balloon. These types of balloons are slightly smaller than the more traditional balloons and dissolve in the stomach by around 4 months.

Discharge from hospital usually occurs on the same day and most people feel well enough to get back to work within a couple of days of the procedure after the discomfort and nausea dies down. On average, people undergoing this type of procedure lose 1.5 to 2 stone (10-12kg). Because the balloon is temporary, it is especially important to adopt healthy lifestyle choices to maintain weight loss in the future.

Reasons to choose or avoid the balloon

People often choose the gastric balloon because it is temporary and avoids the small risks of surgery. The balloon can also be considered in individuals with lower BMIs of 27 kg/m² and above and can also be considered as an initial first to help lose weight in people with extremely high weights (for example if your BMI is greater than 60kg/m²), to reduce the risk of subsequent surgery.

The balloon may not appropriate if you have acid reflux, a hiatus hernia, problems with your oesophagus or if you have a lot of weight to lose. You will not be able to have a balloon if you have had any significant surgery on your stomach before, including previous weight loss surgery.

Potential risks

The gastric balloon is safe, but nonetheless carries some small risks. The following risks are not exhaustive but cover the commonest or most important issues to consider.

The use of a gastroscope has a small risk of infection, bleeding, and perforation of less than 1 in 1000. In the first couple of weeks, the biggest issues that can arise include intolerance of the balloon which results in severe nausea and vomiting. Sometimes these nausea symptoms can last for several weeks. In less than 10% of cases, the gastric balloon will need to be removed earlier than planned. If this occurs, you will usually not be offered a further balloon, however, you should still have access to your aftercare team, including dietitians who will continue to offer nutritional guidance for the length of your after-care programme.

In the medium to longer term, rare complications such as significant ulceration, migration or movement of the balloon into the small bowel can occur. In extremely rare cases, the balloon can cause perforation of the bowel; if this happens, emergency surgery is usually required to treat this. The risk of any of these complications resulting in death is extremely rare and in the order of less than 1 in 10000.

Other considerations

As a procedure which results in significant dietary restriction, it is vitally important to adhere to the post-operative recommendations with respect to medication and other advice that will support your health. You will be required to take anti-acid medication for the duration of the gastric balloon to reduce the risk of ulceration. Very rarely, it may not be possible to place the balloon if an ulcer or other previously undiagnosed conditions of the stomach are identified at the time. In these cases, further tests may be required or alternative approaches to weight loss will need to be discussed.

Novel treatments

Due to the significant problem of obesity, there has always been great interest in finding new approaches which reduce risks and improve outcomes for patients in both the short and long-term. Over the years many contenders in the form of medications, surgical procedures and medical devices have attempted to take their place at the table, but very few have stayed the course. In this section, we'll discuss some of the most recent approaches to managing obesity.

Newer surgical procedures

Newer surgical procedures include the SADI-S (Single Anastomosis Duodenal-Ileal bypass with Sleeve), which is a more extensive type of procedure that combines a sleeve gastrectomy with a type of bypass. Despite some encouraging early results, the SADI-S is still very much in its early days, is a technically challenging procedure to undertake which has been performed by relatively few surgeons, and very little is known about its long-term results and safety. So, caution must be taken when considering this option if it is made available to you by your surgical team.

Robotic surgery is another example of a novel approach which may also provide some additional benefit to patients, particularly in revision surgery cases. Robotic surgery platforms are still under the full control of a surgeon but offer greater dexterity to the surgeon and make tasks such as suturing easier. We are also seeing the potential of robotic surgery expand as artificial intelligence is incorporated into systems which may make decision-making easier for surgeons during procedures. However, currently, robotic surgery is expensive and takes a lot longer to perform than standard keyhole (laparoscopic) surgery. In addition, there has yet to be any research which has clearly shown a definite benefit of robotic surgery over more established laparoscopic approaches.

Endoscopic treatments

More recently, there has been significant interest in endoscopic treatments – such as the endoscopic sleeve gastroplasty or ESG - which takes inspiration from more established procedures but avoids the need for abdominal incisions. These procedures have been made possible due to recent developments in medical devices that allow internal suturing using an endoscopic device. Whilst initial studies suggest that the procedure is safe in the hands of highly skilled and experienced specialists, it is yet to be widely adopted, and very little is known about its long-term effectiveness and future risks of complications.

Undoubtedly the field of endoscopic treatments will continue to grow and play an important role in the treatment of obesity. And whilst it may not take the place of more effective surgical treatments, it may at the very least offer a safe alternative to those looking to avoid surgery.

Regardless of whether you are considering a newer procedure for weight loss, the principles on which informed decision making which we covered elsewhere, remain the same. These include making sure you undertake your own research, speaking to more than one weight loss provider and asking the important questions about risks and complications.

Chapter 4: Surgical weight loss procedures

What is covered in this chapter?

- Sleeve gastrectomy.
- Full or roux-en-y gastric bypass.
- Mini or one/single anastomosis gastric bypass.
- Adjustable gastric band.

Introduction

Now that we have discussed non-surgical options for weight loss, let's now explore the surgical options, describe how they work, discuss risks of complications specific to the procedure and cover reasons to consider them as a choice for weight loss.

The Sleeve Gastrectomy

What is it and how does it work?

The sleeve gastrectomy or gastric sleeve is a permanent procedure which involves removing part of the stomach, leaving it smaller and narrower. It works in three ways:

1. Firstly, because the stomach is smaller, the amount of food and drink that can be consumed is heavily restricted, reducing portion size and making you feel fuller more quickly.
2. Secondly, the part of the stomach removed is responsible for producing a hormone called Ghrelin which causes hunger; by removing this, appetite is usually suppressed.
3. Finally, we also see extremely powerful changes to hormonal signalling pathways which regulate metabolism. In other words, your metabolism increases which allows you to burn off more energy stored as fat.

Smaller portion sizes, suppressed appetite, and an increased metabolism in addition to making the necessary lifestyle choices, are a powerful combination which results in significant and sustained weight loss.

The sleeve gastrectomy started out as the first stage of a two-stage weight loss procedure called the duodenal switch (DS). It wasn't until the late 1990's that it became a standalone procedure. Over time, the technique used to perform the sleeve gastrectomy has been modified and refined resulting in much improved outcomes for patients. Currently, the sleeve is the most popular weight loss procedure undertaken worldwide.

How is it performed?

The procedure is carried out using a keyhole or laparoscopic approach usually using 4 or 5 very small incisions positioned around the upper half of the abdominal wall. A general anaesthetic is required (so you are fast asleep during the procedure), and it takes on average between 30-60 minutes to complete.

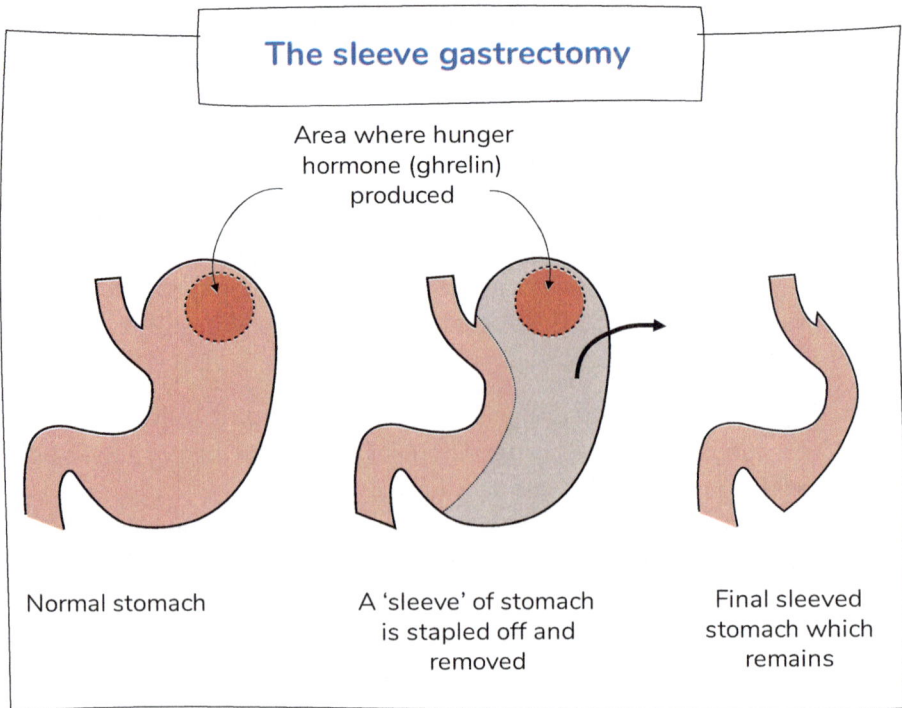

The sleeve gastrectomy

Area where hunger hormone (ghrelin) produced

Normal stomach

A 'sleeve' of stomach is stapled off and removed

Final sleeved stomach which remains

The sleeve is created by using a specialised stapling device which simultaneously seals and cuts the stomach leaving it with a long, narrow shape. This process is guided by temporarily placing a long tube into the stomach during the procedure. Finally, the part of the stomach which is permanently removed is extracted through one of the small incisions. The staples used during the procedure are very small and made of titanium. Titanium is strong, non-magnetic, and well-tolerated by the human body. It is compatible with scanning machines including MRI and extremely unlikely to cause reactions.

I am frequently asked about how much stomach is taken away; is it 70%, 75% or 80%? The short answer is 'it depends'. Everyone will usually end up with a similar size stomach after the procedure as the technique for forming the sleeve gastrectomy is standardised. It results in a stomach which is small enough to cause restriction in eating, but not so small that you are unable to take in enough nutrition. So, if you are starting out with a much bigger stomach than most, more will need to be taken away compared to someone who has a smaller stomach.

Most people can be discharged home the day after surgery by which time you will be able to care for yourself and move freely. Pain and discomfort from the incisions and the carbon dioxide gas used to inflate the abdomen during surgery usually lasts no more than a few days. Physical recovery usually takes between 10 days to 2 weeks by which time you can return to work. Whilst the amount of weight you can expect to lose will be dependent on many factors, on average, people undergoing the sleeve gastrectomy lose three quarters of the extra weight they are carrying by about 12 months after their procedure.

Reasons to choose and avoid the gastric sleeve

People often choose the sleeve because it is a relatively straightforward operation to undertake, it results in significant and sustainable weight loss, and it has fewer short and longer-term issues that we sometimes see with the bypass. The sleeve gastrectomy is particularly effective against metabolic and cardiovascular diseases such as diabetes and high blood pressure. In some cases, especially in situations where patients are very heavy, the sleeve may be used as the first stage in a multi-staged approach to weight loss which may be followed by a gastric bypass.

57

If you have heartburn or acid reflux, or you have other conditions which affect the food pipe or oesophagus (including Barrett's oesophagus), the sleeve may not be a good choice.

Potential Risks

The sleeve gastrectomy is safe, but nonetheless carries some small risks. The following risks are not exhaustive but cover the commonest or most important issues to consider.

As with any operation, there are anaesthetic and general surgical risks such as bleeding, unintentional damage to nearby structures, deep vein thrombosis and pulmonary embolism (blood clots to the legs and lungs) and infection. Significant measures are put in place to reduce the risks of these from happening. In addition, the sleeve gastrectomy carries a small risk (usually less than 1%) of leak, where the staple line does not heal properly. If this happens, you will likely need additional treatment in a specialist hospital which can last several weeks.

In the early days after bariatric surgery, a small number of people struggle with maintaining sufficient nutritional intake which may require readmission to hospital. Sometimes this can be due to strictures or narrowing of the sleeve which require additional attention to manage and treat. The risk of any of these complications resulting in death is extremely rare and in the order of less than 1 in 2000.

In the longer-term, at least 1 in 10 people can develop new symptoms of heartburn and acid reflux. In some cases, this can be severe, impact on quality of life and require conversion to a gastric bypass to alleviate. In a minority of cases, reflux can lead to a pre-cancerous condition called Barrett's oesophagus. The true risk of this is not known but thought to be small. Significant and rapid weight loss can also result in the development of gallstones in approximately 1 in 5 people which may require further surgery to remove the gallbladder if they cause symptoms.

Other considerations

As a procedure which results in significant dietary restriction, it is vitally important to adhere to the post-operative recommendations with respect to supplements and medication that will support your health. You will be required to take lifelong daily multivitamins and supplements such as iron and calcium as well as regular B12 supplementation (which will be covered in greater detail later). Regular blood testing will be required to ensure that your levels are satisfactory. We will discuss this in lots more detail later.

The full (roux-en-y) gastric bypass

What is it and how does it work?

The full or 'roux-en-y' gastric bypass is a procedure which involves making a small pouch from the top of the stomach about the size of a thumb and then joining part of the small intestine to that pouch. This results in food and drink bypassing the bottom part of the stomach and the first part of the intestine. It works in several ways:

- Firstly, because the stomach pouch that receives the food is small, the amount of food and drink that can be consumed is heavily restricted, so that portion sizes are smaller, and you feel fuller more quickly.
- Secondly, your appetite is usually significantly reduced because of changes to the level of circulating hormones responsible for hunger.
- Because food bypasses part of the small intestine (where digested food is usually absorbed), some weight loss is likely to occur because of malabsorption.
- Finally, we also see extremely powerful changes to hormonal signalling pathways which regulate metabolism. In other words, your metabolism increases which allows you to burn off more energy stored as fat.

Smaller portion sizes, suppressed appetite, reduced food absorption, and an increased metabolism in addition to making the necessary lifestyle choices, are a powerful combination which results in significant and sustained weight loss.

The gastric bypass is the most established and longest serving bariatric surgical procedure currently available. It is the gold-standard against which all other procedures are compared. The first type of gastric bypass was undertaken in the 1950s, whilst the roux-en-y or full bypass as we know it today was first developed and performed in the 1960s using open surgery. The 1990's saw the development of laparoscopic or keyhole surgery which resulted in significant reductions in the risks associated with the bypass.

How is it performed?

The procedure is carried out using a keyhole or laparoscopic approach usually using 4 or 5 very small incisions positioned around the upper half of the abdominal wall. A general anaesthetic is required (so you are fast asleep during this procedure), and it takes on average between 1 to 2 hours to complete.

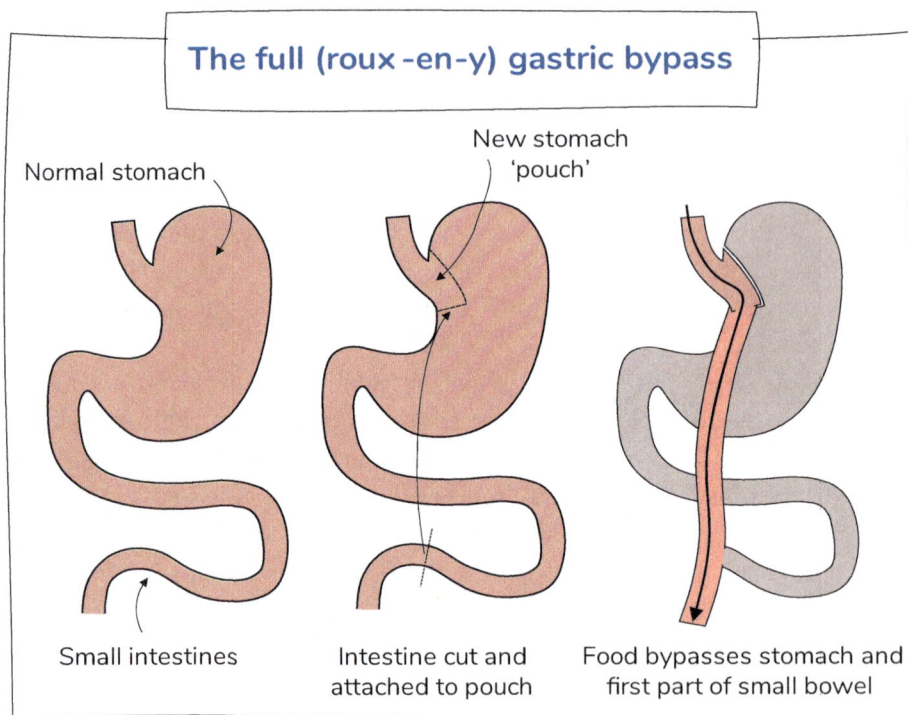

The full (roux -en-y) gastric bypass

Normal stomach

New stomach 'pouch'

Small intestines

Intestine cut and attached to pouch

Food bypasses stomach and first part of small bowel

Much like the sleeve and mini-gastric bypass, the full bypass is undertaken using a specialised stapling device which simultaneously seals and cuts the stomach. A small pouch is made using this device before joining the small intestine to it. A further join between the intestine is also made. These joins are generally completed using a combination of staples and sutures although different techniques can be used by surgeons all of which are perfectly safe. Finally, due to the way that the bypass is created, internal openings need to be closed to reduce the risk of internal hernias in the future.

Most people can be discharged home the day after surgery by which time you will be able to care for yourself and move freely. Pain and discomfort from the incisions and the carbon dioxide gas used to inflate the abdomen during surgery usually lasts no more than a few days. Physical recovery usually takes between 10 days to 2 weeks by which time you can return to work.

Whilst the amount of weight you can expect to lose depends on many factors, on average, people undergoing bypass lose 80% of the extra weight they are carrying by about 12 months after their surgery.

Reasons to choose and avoid the gastric bypass

People often choose the full bypass because it is the most established type of bariatric surgery and therefore the most understood in terms of long-term benefits and downsides. It also results in significant and sustainable weight loss and may better protect against weight-regain in the future compared to other options such as the sleeve or gastric band. The bypass is also the most effective procedure against metabolic and cardiovascular diseases such as diabetes and high blood pressure and may be the preferred option in patients who have well-established heartburn and acid reflux.

The bypass is undoubtedly a more complex operation that involves surgery on the small bowel. Therefore, if you have had significant or previous complex abdominal surgery, the bypass may not be an appropriate option due to pre-existing scar tissue. This may increase the technical challenges of performing it, and therefore increase the risks of complications associated with the procedure. If your BMI is particularly high, the amount of intra-abdominal fat that is seen during surgery may make it technically more challenging to complete. In these circumstances, it may be a better option to consider a mini-bypass or a gastric sleeve.

A previous diagnosis of bowel disorders such as inflammatory bowel disease or functional disorders are another reason to avoid a bypass. In these cases, the bypass can make accessing certain parts of the gastrointestinal tract difficult for future investigations, and in some cases can make symptoms worse. Bypass surgery is also linked to a higher chance of developing Dumping syndrome (a collection of signs and symptoms which includes dramatic changes to blood sugar levels, headache, low blood pressure, vomiting, diarrhoea, abdominal cramps, and sweating) compared to the gastric sleeve. We will explore Dumping Syndrome in greater detail at another point.

Potential risks

The gastric bypass is safe, but nonetheless carries some small risks. The following risks are not exhaustive but cover the commonest or most important issues to consider.

As with any operation, there are anaesthetic and general surgical risks such as bleeding, unintentional damage to nearby structures, deep vein thrombosis, pulmonary embolism (blood clots to the legs and lungs) and infection. Significant measures are put in place to reduce the risks of these from happening. In addition, the bypass carries a small risk (usually less than 1%) of leak, where the staple line or surgical joins do not heal properly. If this happens, you will likely need additional treatment in a specialist hospital which can last several weeks.

In the early days after bariatric surgery, some people struggle with maintaining sufficient nutritional intake which may require readmission to hospital. Sometimes this can be due to strictures or narrowing of the join between the pouch and the bowel, which may require additional treatment to manage and treat. Due to the increased complexity of surgery, there is a slightly higher overall risk of complications compared to other less invasive procedures such as the sleeve. The risk of requiring further treatments is in the order of less than 5% of cases. The risk of any of these complications resulting in death is extremely rare and in the order of less than 1 in 2000.

Because part of the intestine is being bypassed, we see a higher rate of nutritional deficiencies in the case of the gastric bypass compared to the sleeve gastrectomy for example. This highlights the importance of taking lifelong multi-vitamins to reduce the risk of these issues. The bypass is also associated with a chance of developing twists or internal hernias of the bowel due to the way in which the bypass is performed. Whilst steps are taken to reduce the risk of this happening, the risk of this happening can never be completely eliminated. Finally, significant, and rapid weight loss can also result in the development of gallstones in approximately 1 in 5 people which may require further surgery to remove the gallbladder if they cause symptoms.

Other considerations

As a procedure which results in significant dietary restriction, it is vitally important to adhere to the post-operative recommendations with respect to supplements and medication that will support your health. You will be required to take lifelong daily multivitamins and supplements such as iron and calcium as well as regular B12 supplementation (which will be covered in greater detail later). Regular blood testing will be required to ensure that your levels are satisfactory. We will discuss this in lots more detail later.

Very rarely, it may not be possible to undertake the bypass due to several factors including the presence of scar tissue from previous surgery or because the amount of fat inside the abdomen may make it difficult to join the small bowel to the stomach pouch. This may only be discovered at the time of surgery. At this point, a decision will need to be made whether to undertake either a mini-bypass or sleeve versus doing nothing at all. This scenario should be discussed between you and your surgeon before your operation.

Finally, unlike the sleeve, the bypass does not involve permanently removing any part of the stomach from the body. However, it should still be considered as an irreversible procedure. In certain circumstances, it may be necessary to reverse the bypass. However, this is a complex procedure that doesn't return the gastrointestinal tract completely back to its original form.

The 'mini' (or one/single anastomosis) gastric bypass

What is it and how does it work?

The 'mini' gastric bypass is a procedure which involves making a small pouch from the top of the stomach and then joining part of the small intestine to that pouch. This results in food and drink bypassing the bottom part of the stomach and the first part of the intestine. It works in several ways:

- Firstly, because the stomach pouch that receives the food is small, the amount of food and drink that can be consumed is heavily restricted, so that portion sizes are smaller, and you feel fuller more quickly.
- Secondly, your appetite is usually significantly reduced because of changes to the level of circulating hormones responsible for hunger.
- Because food bypasses part of the small intestine (where digested food is usually absorbed), some weight loss is likely to occur because of malabsorption.
- Finally, we also see extremely powerful changes to hormonal signalling pathways which regulate metabolism. In other words, your

metabolism increases which allows you to burn off more energy stored as fat.

Smaller portion sizes, suppressed appetite, reduced food absorption, and an increased metabolism in addition to making the necessary lifestyle choices, are a powerful combination which results in significant and sustained weight loss.

The mini gastric bypass was developed in the late 1990s to reduce the technical challenges and operating times that surgeons are sometimes faced with when performing the full gastric bypass. It was named the 'mini' bypass because it is more straightforward to perform and not because the resulting weight loss or impacts on health are inferior to the 'full' bypass; in fact, some research studies suggest that weight loss may even be superior. Over the last 5 to 10 years, it has certainly become more established in wider surgical practice across the world and whilst initial results seem to be very similar to those of the full bypass, longer-term real-world data is still being collected.

How is it performed?

The procedure is carried out using a keyhole or laparoscopic approach usually using 4 or 5 very small incisions positioned around the upper half of the abdominal wall. A general anaesthetic is required (so you are fast asleep during this procedure), and it takes on average between 45 to 90 minutes to complete.

Much like the sleeve and full bypass, the mini bypass is undertaken using a specialised stapling device which simultaneously seals and cuts the stomach. Compared to the full bypass, the stomach pouch is longer and there is only one surgical join (made between the small intestine and the pouch) compared to the two joins in the full bypass. As with the full bypass, the join between the intestine and the pouch is generally completed using a combination of staples and sutures although different techniques can be used by surgeons all of which are perfectly safe. Finally, due to the way that the mini bypass is created, an internal opening need to be closed to reduce the risk of internal hernias in the future.

Most people can be discharged home the day after surgery by which time you will be able to care for yourself and move freely. Pain and discomfort from the incisions and the carbon dioxide gas used to inflate the abdomen during surgery usually lasts no more than a few days. Physical recovery usually takes between 10 days to 2 weeks by which time you can return to work.

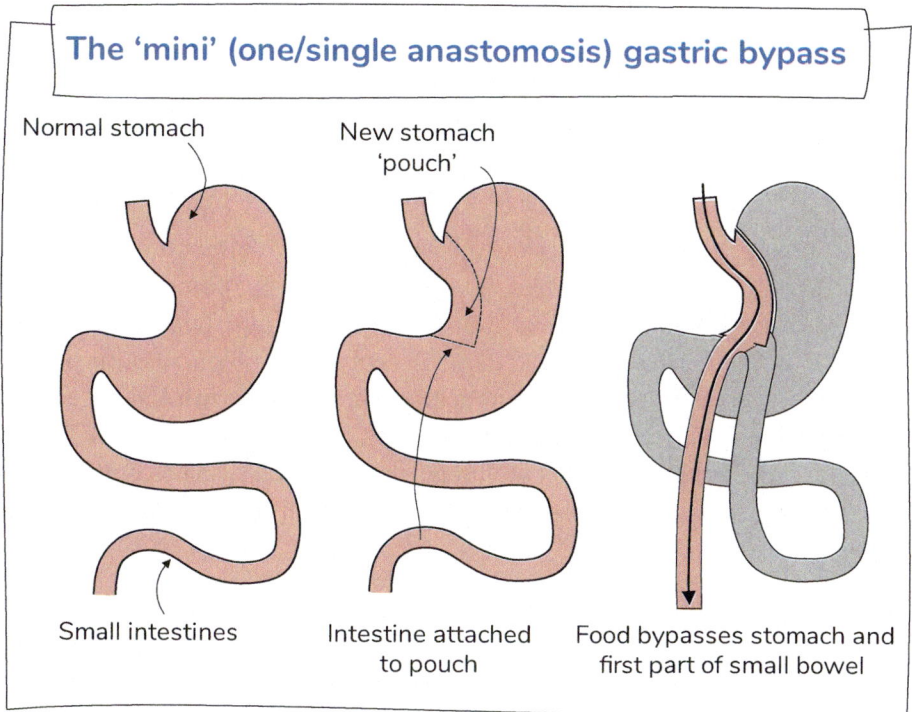

The 'mini' (one/single anastomosis) gastric bypass

Normal stomach

New stomach 'pouch'

Small intestines

Intestine attached to pouch

Food bypasses stomach and first part of small bowel

Whilst the amount of weight you can expect to lose will be dependent on many factors, on average, people undergoing the mini bypass lose 80% of the extra weight they are carrying by about 12 months after surgery. This is very similar to results from the full bypass and underlines the fact that the term 'mini' refers to the technical aspects of performing the operation and not to its weight loss results.

Reasons to choose and avoid the mini bypass

People often choose the mini bypass because it seems to offer similar results to the full bypass, but as this operation is less technically demanding, the short-term risks are likely to be smaller. If you are older or very heavy and need a bypass type procedure, then the mini-bypass may be a better option compared to the full bypass, again because it is less technically demanding to perform. The mini bypass results in significant and sustainable weight loss and it may better protect against weight-regain in the future compared to other options such as the sleeve or gastric band. Finally, the mini bypass is highly effective against metabolic and cardiovascular diseases such as diabetes and high blood pressure.

The main issue with the mini-bypass certainly compared to the full bypass is the lack of long-term 'real-world' data with respect to results and side effects. Whilst the initial short- and medium-term data suggests good results, I am personally more cautious about offering the mini-bypass to younger patients.

The mini bypass is a complex operation that involves surgery on the bowel. Therefore, if you have had significant or previous complex abdominal surgery, the bypass may not be an appropriate option due to pre-existing scar tissue. This may increase the technical challenges of performing it, and therefore increase the risks of complications associated with the procedure. If your weight is particularly high, the amount of intra-abdominal fat that we see during surgery may make it technically more challenging to complete. In these circumstances, it may be a better option to consider a sleeve gastrectomy.

A previous diagnosis of bowel disorders such as inflammatory bowel disease or functional disorders are another reason to avoid a bypass. In these cases, the mini bypass can make accessing certain parts of the gastrointestinal tract difficult for future investigations and in some cases can make symptoms worse. The mini-bypass surgery is linked to a higher chance of developing Dumping syndrome (a collection of signs and symptoms which includes dramatic changes to blood sugar levels, headache, low blood pressure, vomiting, diarrhoea, abdominal cramps, and sweating) compared to the gastric sleeve. We will explore Dumping Syndrome in greater detail at another point.

Potential risks

The mini bypass is safe, but nonetheless carries some small risks. The following risks are not exhaustive but cover the commonest or most important issues to consider.

As with any operation, there are anaesthetic and general surgical risks such as bleeding, unintentional damage to nearby structures, deep vein thrombosis, pulmonary embolism (blood clots to the legs and lungs) and infection. Significant measures are put in place to reduce the risks of these from happening. In addition, the bypass carries a small risk (usually less than 1%) of leak, where the staple line or surgical joins do not heal properly. If this happens, you will likely need additional treatment in a specialist hospital which can last several weeks.

In the early days after bariatric surgery, some people struggle with maintaining sufficient nutritional intake which may require readmission to hospital. Sometimes this can be due to strictures or narrowing of the join between the pouch and the bowel, which may require additional treatment to manage and treat. Due to the increased complexity of surgery, there is a slightly higher overall risk of complications compared to other less invasive procedures such as the sleeve. The risk of requiring further treatments is in the order of less than 5% of cases. The risk of any of these complications resulting in death is extremely rare and in the order of less than 1 in 2000.

Because part of the intestine is being bypassed, we see a higher rate of nutritional deficiencies in the case of the gastric bypass compared to the sleeve gastrectomy for example. This highlights the importance of taking lifelong multi-vitamins to reduce the risk of these issues. The mini bypass is also associated with a chance of developing twists or internal hernias of the bowel due to the way in which the bypass is performed. Whilst steps are taken to reduce the risk of this happening, the risk of this happening can never be completely eliminated.

Bile reflux is a particularly unique issue related to the mini bypass. This occurs when bile, produced by the liver, travels into the small bowel, into the gastric pouch and in some case can reflux backwards up the stomach pouch and into the oesophagus (also known as the gullet or food pipe). Symptoms of bile reflux can mimic heartburn, and in some cases can lead to unrelenting and severe pain and reflux. Whilst the risk of this seems to be small, it can be more difficult to treat and, in some cases, requires further surgery to convert the mini-bypass to a full roux-en-y bypass.

Finally, significant, and rapid weight loss can also result in the development of gallstones in approximately 1 in 5 people which may require further surgery to remove the gallbladder if they cause symptoms.

Other considerations

As a procedure which results in significant dietary restriction, it is vitally important to adhere to the post-operative recommendations with respect to supplements and medication that will support your health. You will be required to take lifelong daily multivitamins and supplements such as iron and calcium as well as regular B12 supplementation (which will be covered in greater detail later). Regular blood testing will be required to ensure that your levels are satisfactory. We will discuss this in lots more detail later.

Very rarely, it may not be possible to undertake the mini bypass due to several factors including the presence of scar tissue from previous surgery or because the amount of fat inside the abdomen may make it difficult to join the small bowel to the stomach pouch. This may only be discovered at the time of surgery. At this point, a decision will need to be made whether to undertake a gastric sleeve versus doing nothing at all. This scenario should be discussed between you and your surgeon before your operation.

Finally, unlike the sleeve, the mini bypass does not involve permanently removing any part of the stomach from the body. However, it should still be considered as an irreversible procedure. In certain circumstances, it may be necessary to reverse the mini bypass. However, this is a complex procedure that doesn't return the gastrointestinal tract completely back to its original form.

The gastric band

What is it and how does it work?

The gastric band is an adjustable silicone ring which is placed around the top of the stomach. The band is connected by a long narrow tube to a port which is fixed to the abdominal wall muscles deep to the skin. This port allows fluid to be introduced into and removed from the gastric band by a specialist which alters the degree of restriction the band provides. By increasing the amount of fluid and restriction the band offers, patients find that they feel fuller more quickly. This is thought to be due to stimulation of nerve pathways between the top of the stomach to the brain. The band does not address underlying hormonally mediated hunger sensations unlike the sleeve gastrectomy or gastric bypass.

The first non-adjustable gastric band was placed in the late 1970s after which developments were made to produce an adjustable version in the 1980s. The 1990's saw the first laparoscopically inserted gastric band inserted, but it wasn't until the late 90s and early 2000's that the band became widely popular as an alternative to the gastric bypass. In the late 2000's the popularity of the band began to decline rapidly due to the wider adoption of the sleeve gastrectomy and the increased incidence of problems linked to the band.

How is it performed?

The procedure is carried out using a keyhole or laparoscopic approach usually using 4 or 5 very small incisions positioned around the upper half of the abdominal wall. A general anaesthetic is required (so you are fast asleep during the procedure), and it takes on average between 30-60 minutes to complete. Bands come in different sizes. Once an assessment has been made with respect to which band size is most appropriate, it is placed into position. Additional sutures are then placed to reduce the chance of the band moving. The tubing is attached to the adjustment port, which is then secured to the muscular layer of the abdominal wall.

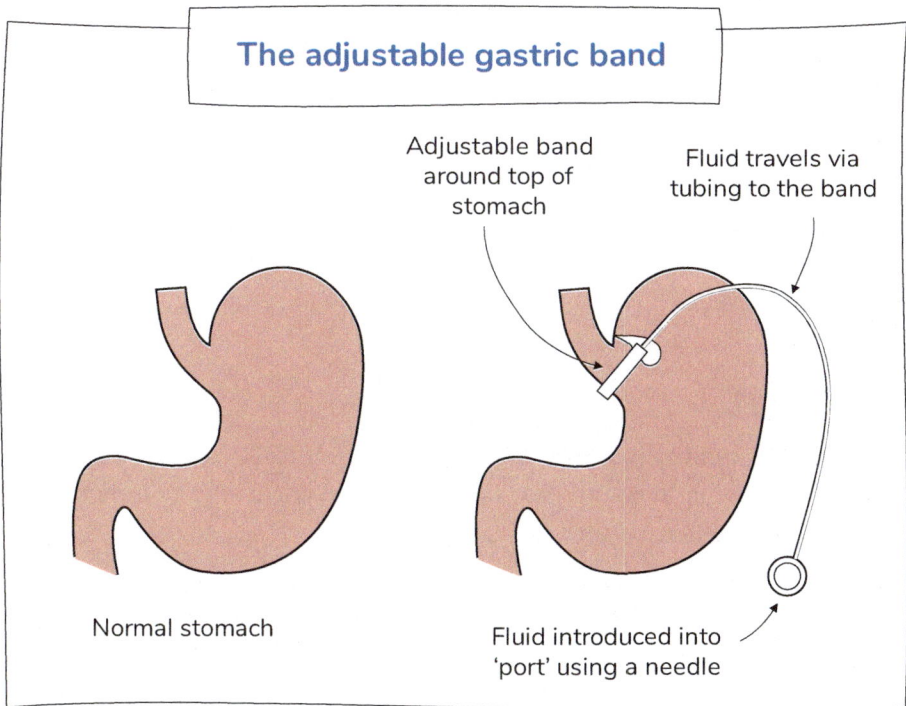

The adjustable gastric band

Adjustable band around top of stomach

Fluid travels via tubing to the band

Normal stomach

Fluid introduced into 'port' using a needle

At the time of surgery, it is my practice to place a minimal amount of fluid to prime the band, without it resulting in any significant restriction. This is done to reduce the risk of acute problems with vomiting in the first few weeks after surgery. The first band fill is usually undertaken at 6 weeks following surgery. Each surgeon's practice may vary slightly, and so discussions about initial band fills should be had with your surgeon before surgery.

Most people can be discharged either on the same day or the day after surgery, by which time you be able to care for yourself and move freely. Pain and discomfort from the incisions and the carbon dioxide gas used to inflate the abdomen during surgery usually lasts no more than a few days. Physical recovery usually takes between 10 days to 2 weeks by which time you can return to work.

Whilst the amount of weight you can expect to lose will be dependent on many factors, on average, people undergoing the gastric band lose 50% of the extra weight they are carrying by about 12 months after surgery.

Reasons to choose and avoid the gastric band

People often choose the band because it is a relatively straightforward operation to undertake and it is potentially reversible.

If you have acid heartburn or reflux, have other conditions which affect the oesophagus, or if your BMI is particularly high, the band may not be a good choice. We are also becoming more aware of a growing significant number of patients who are having to undergo revision surgery to remove their band. Consequently, for many the band is no longer seen as a long-term tool.

Potential risks

The band is generally a safe option, but nonetheless carries some small risks. The following risks are not exhaustive but cover the commonest or most important issues to consider.

As with any operation, there are anaesthetic and general surgical risks such as bleeding, unintentional damage to nearby structures, deep vein thrombosis, pulmonary embolism (blood clots to the legs and lungs) and infection. Significant measures are put in place to reduce the risks of these from happening. As with any surgical operation, there are anaesthetic and general surgical risks such as bleeding, unintentional damage to nearby structures, deep vein thrombosis, pulmonary embolism (or blood clots to the legs and lungs) and infection. Significant measures are put in place to reduce the risks of these from happening. The risk of any of these complications resulting in death is extremely rare.

In the early days after gastric band surgery, some people struggle with maintaining sufficient nutritional intake which may require readmission to hospital. In the longer-term, the gastric band can be associated with infection, slippage – where the stomach slips through the band, erosion into the stomach and the development of stricture and blockages which can manifest as vomiting and acid reflux. Sometimes band slippage can occur soon after surgery.

Some of these problems can present suddenly, requiring urgent admission to hospital and further surgery to correct. In my experience, once more chronic problems become established, it can be challenging to put them right, and usually surgery to remove the band is required. At any point, there is a small risk of malfunction of the band, such as leakage, fracture or detachment of the tubing and flipping of the adjustment port. All of these would render the band ineffective and would likely need corrective surgery to put right. In this scenario, the band or part of it can sometimes be replaced, but it is common that the band needs to be removed entirely if these problems occur. Problems which may need the band removed are covered later in this book.

Finally, as with all other surgical options, significant and rapid weight loss can also result in the development of gallstones in approximately 1 in 5 people which may require further surgery to remove the gallbladder if they cause symptoms.

Other considerations

As a procedure which results in significant dietary restriction, it is vitally important to adhere to the post-operative recommendations with respect to supplements and medication that will support your health.

Very rarely, it may not be possible to fit the band due to several factors including the presence of scar tissue from previous surgery or excessive amounts of fat that makes it technically challenging to place the band. This may only be discovered at the time of surgery and would mean that the procedure would not go ahead as planned.

Importantly, regular adjustments of the band are required in the first 12 months after surgery. The aim is to allow the band to provide sufficient

71

dietary restriction without it being too tight. We often use a traffic light system to help us understand how much restriction is being provided; yellow means too loose, red means too tight and green means just right. Where this balance lies differs for everyone and can be challenging in some to get right. Ensuring that the band is not too tight is important as this can lead to chronic dilatation of the portion of stomach above the band (pouch dilatation). If this occurs, it is usually necessary to deflate the band, give the stomach an opportunity to recover, and start over with respect to the band filling process. There are additional logistical considerations which need to be planned in relation to where these band adjustments will take place. Some clinics may require you to travel significant distances for adjustments which will need to be factored in around a busy work or life schedule.

Finally, there may be specific circumstances where extra caution is required with respect to your band. In some cases, patients can have higher levels of restriction during and shortly after flying. Consequently, it may be helpful to have some fluid removed before a flight. Similarly, during pregnancy, it is a good idea to deflate band to ensure that vomiting isn't made worse and that both mother and baby are able to get the required nutrients to support a healthy pregnancy.

Chapter 5: Revision procedures and surgery

What is covered in this chapter?

- Reasons why revision surgery may be required.
- Potential risks and results.
- Types of revision procedures.

Introduction

This section is aimed at those who are facing challenges after primary or first-time weight loss surgery and are considering 'revision surgery'. 'Revision surgery' is the term used for any additional operation which is needed after a weight loss procedure. However, this chapter is also important for those considering surgery the first time round. Understanding the reasons why revision surgery may be required in the future will give you a better understanding of some of the challenges and pitfalls that a small proportion of people may face and allow you to make more informed decisions.

There are several reasons why it may be appropriate or necessary to consider revision surgery. The commonest include:

- To correct complications both in the immediate period after surgery and in the longer-term
- Or to partly address inadequate weight loss or weight-regain

Revision surgery is a complex area which requires careful work-up by an experienced team of specialists, which can include doctors, nurses, dietitians, and psychologists. If you are considering revision surgery, it is important to ensure the surgeon and team looking after you are experienced in this field and can help you navigate through nuances and further investigations required during the decision-making process.

Rates of revision surgery

The rate at which revision surgery is needed depends on many factors including those related to the patient (such as the degree to which post-operative recommendations and healthy lifestyle choices are adopted), the type of surgery which has originally been undertaken (we know that a growing number of patients with the gastric band are requiring its removal), and the experience of the surgeon performing the original surgery (particularly if inexperience has resulted in an avoidable complication). Current estimates suggest that up to 60% of gastric bands will need revision surgery compared to the gastric sleeve and bypass which may require revision surgery in around 5-10% of cases.

Workup & Investigations

It is often necessary to undertake several carefully planned investigations to determine whether further surgery is either needed or appropriate. The types of investigations required depends very much on the problem which the patient has presented with. Tests may include X-rays such as a barium swallow or a gastroscopy (camera test sometimes referred to as endoscopy). Occasionally it is necessary to undertake further diagnostic surgical procedures such as a laparoscopy to get to the bottom of the issue and understand the role that further surgery may provide.

Risks and Complications

If deemed appropriate, it is important to keep in mind that revision surgery remains safe and effective, and the risks associated with it are small. However, compared to primary or 'first-time' surgery, the risks of developing certain complications are slightly higher. In addition to the risks of the procedure being carried out (which have been covered elsewhere) there is also a slightly higher chance of poor healing and leaks from the staple lines or surgical joins which can require additional treatments including a return to the operating theatre and prolonged stays in hospital. Due to the unpredictability of revision surgery, it may be necessary to change the agreed surgical plan during the operation. In some cases, it may not be possible to undertake any type of revision weight loss surgery at all.

Results from revision surgery

Without doubt, the best opportunity to maximise and sustain weight loss in the long-term is following first time surgery. This highlights the importance of investing the time to make the right decisions from the outset. Weight loss results from revision surgery can be less predictable for many reasons:

1. Scar tissue: Revision surgery is more complex because of scarring or thickened tissue from previous surgery. This thickened scar tissue can make it difficult for surgeons to easily manipulate the stomach and intestines to size the sleeve and bypass for example, as they would usually be able to during first time surgery. This may be the case during conversion from a gastric band to a sleeve or a gastric bypass.

2. Anatomical changes: After first time bariatric surgery, the anatomy of the stomach and intestines is altered, which may make subsequent procedures more difficult to perform. To ensure the risks of revision surgery are minimised, the surgeon may need to modify the planned approach to account for these changes, which can affect weight loss outcomes.

3. Pre-existing conditions: Patients who undergo revision bariatric surgery often have pre-existing health conditions, such as diabetes or heart disease, which require medications which can affect the ability to lose weight. Some of these same conditions may also make it more challenging to perform revision surgery.

4. Adherence to post-operative recommendations: If revision surgery is being considered because of weight regain, it is especially important to understand how this occurred to reduce the risk of it happening again in the future. This often means that additional and more robust strategies to address triggers to eating or food seeking behaviours are required, and other underlying factors are properly addressed. The topic of weight loss and weight regain will be covered in greater detail later.

Why does revision surgery cost more?

The cost of revision surgery reflects the complexity and the additional operating time required compared to primary or 'first-time' surgery. Revision surgery may also require a longer stay in hospital, the need for high dependency unit (HDU) care, different post-operative medications, specific blood tests and other investigations. These factors will impact on cost which cannot be compared to primary surgery. For example, converting a band to a sleeve gastrectomy will cost more than a first-time sleeve gastrectomy because of the additional time it takes to remove the band, tube and adjustment port, take down the inevitable thickened scar tissue, and making an assessment as to whether it is safe to proceed. At that point, a sleeve gastrectomy could be performed, which in some cases may require us to use additional tissues reinforcement technology to reduce the risk of staple line leaks. There may be other unexpected findings such as the repair of a hiatus hernia (covered in more detail later) which may be more complicated to perform again because of the presence of scar tissue. This example underpins the complexity of these procedures and why they should be undertaken by teams with the appropriate experience.

Revision surgery related to the gastric band

In addition to inadequate weight loss and weight-regain, common reasons for requiring revision surgery following a gastric band include:

- Slippage of the band where the stomach slides up through the gastric band causing a blockage and vomiting.
- Erosion into the stomach which can be a very serious and challenging problem to manage.
- Infection of any part of the gastric band including the port, tubing, the adjustable part around the stomach all of which can lead to internal infections.
- Development of acid reflux or difficulties with swallowing or food sticking.
- Vomiting, regurgitation, and persistent nausea.
- Chronic pain.
- Problems with the band adjustment port such as flipping or movement.
- Malfunction such as fractures or leakage of the band

Removal of the gastric band

After the necessary investigations have been undertaken and fluid completely removed from the band, often the most straightforward approach to relieving many of these issues is to remove the gastric band altogether.

Depending on the underlying reason, this is often a relatively straightforward procedure which takes between 30 to 45 minutes to complete, although it can take longer if the band has eroded into the stomach or caused other serious complications. The procedure is undertaken laparoscopically (using small keyhole incisions) under a general anaesthetic although there is a very small potential for conversion to open surgery (in less than 1 in every 1000 cases). 'Problem' bands can sometimes result in unexpected findings that will need to be managed at the time. For example, dense scarring from a previously undiagnosed infection or erosion will lengthen the procedure time and may need you to stay in hospital for longer. Assuming a relatively straightforward procedure, most people can go home on the same day of surgery and return to full activity within 10-14 days of surgery.

As with any surgical operation, there are anaesthetic and general surgical risks such as bleeding, unintentional damage to nearby structures, deep vein thrombosis, pulmonary embolism (or blood clots to the legs and lungs) and infection. Significant measures are put in place to reduce the risks of these from happening. Because of the varying types of bands used in patients over the years, and the length of time some of these bands have been in place, there is a small chance that parts of the band may have partly disintegrated or be unknowingly left behind inside the abdomen or within the abdominal wall. Great care is taken to minimise this risk, including careful examination of the entire band after it is removed.

Further surgery after the band

Often, people who have had some success with the band or have regained weight, wish to consider alternative procedures. Both the sleeve gastrectomy and gastric bypass are procedures which may be undertaken in this scenario, although there are many factors which need to be taken into consideration when deciding which options are most suitable.

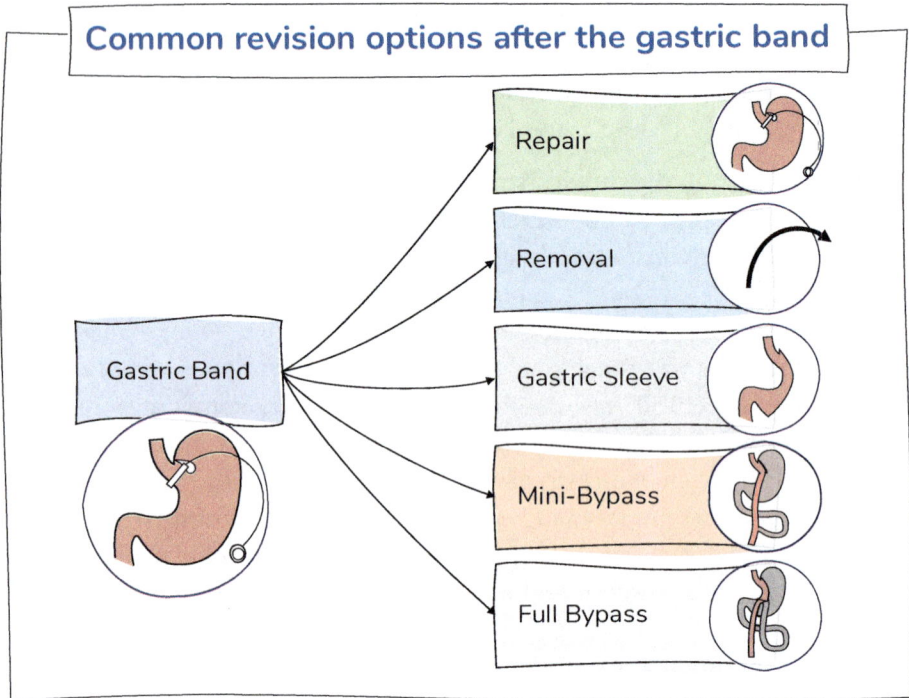

Common revision options after the gastric band

Gastric Band

Repair

Removal

Gastric Sleeve

Mini-Bypass

Full Bypass

For example, if a band has resulted in significant damage to the function of the oesophagus or is associated with significant acid reflux, then it is likely that the sleeve gastrectomy would not be an appropriate option. If the band has caused a serious infection which may have resulted in significant abdominal adhesions or scar tissue for example, then the bypass may not be safe to undertake.

The other consideration is whether to undertake gastric band revision surgery using a single or multi-staged approach. Sometimes it is possible to remove the band and convert to another procedure at the same time, whereas other times it is more appropriate to remove the band, allow any adhesions, swelling or inflammation to settle down, before proceeding to either a sleeve or bypass. Even if a single stage approach is planned, there is no guarantee that this can be performed until after careful assessment is made at the time of surgery.

Revision surgery following a sleeve gastrectomy

In addition to inadequate weight loss and weight-regain, common reasons for requiring revision surgery following a sleeve gastrectomy include:

- Managing complications such as leaks (or non-healing) of the staple line
- strictures or deformity (or a tight narrowing of the stomach)
- Significant stretching or dilatation of the sleeve
- and development of significant acid reflux symptoms

Leaks following sleeve surgery are thankfully rare. However, if this occurs, further treatment in the acute or emergency setting will usually be required. The management of leaks is a complex area that is outside the scope of this book, but treatment usually takes the form of further procedures at a specialist hospital which can last several weeks.

Strictures or narrowing of the sleeve can sometimes occur particularly if the sleeve has been made too tight. A narrowing of the sleeve can also occur if the staple line becomes twisted. It may be necessary to undertake procedures to stretch the sleeve in this scenario. This involves using a gastroscope also known as an endoscopy or camera to guide a small inflatable balloon into the sleeve where it is used to stretch open the narrowing. Sometimes, this may not be successful, and the sleeve requires conversion to a bypass procedure.

A sensation of inadequate restriction may sometimes be due to dilatation or stretching of the sleeve. Some surgeons may suggest a re-sleeve in cases of significant dilatations, but this rarely results in significant and sustained weight loss in the long-term. Often a more appropriate surgical approach would be to consider a bypass in this scenario.

Up to 10-15% of people may develop new symptoms of acid reflux after a sleeve. Often this can be controlled by medication or a change in diet. Sometimes a diagnosis of hiatus hernia is made which, if repaired, can improve symptoms significantly. As a last resort, where symptoms of reflux are so severe that they affect quality of life, conversion to a full bypass may be necessary. This is thought to be required in around 3% of cases.

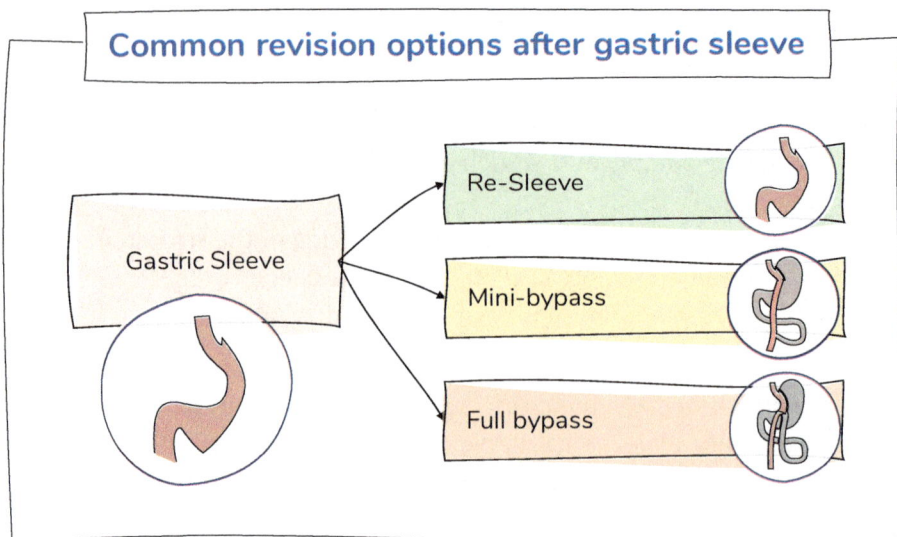

Common revision options after gastric sleeve

Gastric Sleeve

Re-Sleeve

Mini-bypass

Full bypass

Both the full and mini-gastric bypasses are procedures which may be suitable to address weight-regain following a gastric sleeve. Newer, more invasive procedures (including the SADI-S - single anastomosis duodenal-ileal bypass with sleeve), may also be considered by experienced surgical practices. Their suitability and appropriateness need to be carefully discussed by consultation with an experienced surgeon, and with the support of a multi-disciplinary team of healthcare professionals to address risk factors which may have contributed to weight regain. As with any revision procedure, careful assessment at the time of surgery is required to ensure it is safe to proceed.

Revision surgery following a gastric bypass

As the bypass is a more invasive procedure, it is inevitable that it is associated with a different profile of revision surgery than the sleeve gastrectomy and gastric band. In addition to inadequate weight loss and weight-regain, common reasons for revision surgery after a gastric bypass include:

- Strictures (or a tight narrowing of the join between the stomach and bowel)
- Bowel obstruction or blockage – due to scarring or internal hernias
- Chronic stomach ulcers and inflammation of the pouch

- Excessive weight loss or nutritional deficiency
- Severe Dumping syndrome
- And in the case of the mini-bypass, bile reflux

Strictures or narrowing can occur at the surgical joins between the stomach and the bowel or in the case of the full bypass, at the second surgical join between the two parts of the intestine known as the jejuno-jejunostomy (or 'JJ' for short). Sometimes this can be managed using a gastroscope (also known as an endoscopy or camera test) to guide down a balloon where it is used to stretch open the narrowing. If this is unsuccessful, then further surgery to revise the joins may be required.

Bowel obstruction is a rare but serious complication of gastric bypass surgery. This may happen due to scarring or adhesions, and sometimes can occur if the bowel twists on itself through an internal hernia. If a patient develops a blockage in their digestive system, revision surgery may be necessary to alleviate the obstruction. This may present chronically as intermittent abdominal pain, or as an emergency with severe abdominal pain and vomiting.

Ulcers can cause pain, bleeding, and perforation of the stomach lining. If a patient develops an ulcer, revision surgery may be necessary to remove the ulcer and prevent further complications.

Rarely, bypass surgery can result in too much weight loss. Nutritional deficiencies can occur, particularly if there has been poor compliance with taking multivitamins and supplements. Whilst most of the time these scenarios can be managed by correcting deficiencies through nutritional support, in rare circumstances it may be necessary to reverse the gastric bypass. This is a complex procedure that doesn't return the gastrointestinal tract entirely back to its original form.

Dumping syndrome is a group of symptoms that can occur particularly after eating high-sugar or high-carbohydrate foods. This occurs more so with bypass surgery than the sleeve. Whilst these symptoms can often be controlled by following strict dietary advice or in some cases medications, very rarely, Dumping syndrome can be so severe that reversal of the bypass may be required. We will discuss Dumping Syndrome in greater detail later.

Bile reflux is a condition in which bile produced by the liver flows back into the stomach pouch and into the oesophagus (also known as the gullet or food-pipe). This is more likely with a mini bypass than with a full bypass due to the way in which the bowel is joined to the stomach pouch. Symptoms can mimic acid reflux, but these can typically be more severe and sometimes challenging to treat. In rare occasions, it may be necessary to revise the bypass and even convert a mini bypass to a full bypass to better manage symptoms.

Like in the case of the sleeve gastrectomy, some patients may not achieve their desired weight loss or may experience weight regain after gastric bypass surgery. Patients may feel less restriction than before, and this may be due to several causes including quicker emptying of the stomach pouch or an increased food capacity of the stomach and the small intestine. There are several possibilities that can be considered in this scenario, such as endoscopic suturing of the join between the pouch and the intestine (called the TORe or 'Stomaphyx'), surgical revision of the gastric pouch or even changing the total length of the bypass.

It is important to note that revision surgery following gastric bypass surgery is usually considered a last resort after other options have been exhausted, as this rarely results in the outcomes that patients which to achieve.

Artificial feeding after surgery

In some circumstances - particularly if there has been a complication related to surgery - your team will need to think carefully about how to help you maintain sufficient levels of nutrition. This helps support the healing process and ensures that weight loss is not excessive. In the extremely rare scenario where you are unable to (or not allowed to) eat and drink (for example if you have been diagnosed with a leak, a narrowing, or a stricture), other routes of nutrition will need to be considered.

TPN (total parenteral nutrition)

Total parental nutrition (or TPN) involves placing liquid feed directly into a vein in your hand or arm through a cannula (intravenous drip). In some cases, a special type of intravenous line will need to be inserted (called a PICC line) to deliver this type of feed. TPN is commonly used either in the short term whilst further tests are being carried out, in scenarios where it is not possible to introduce food into the intestine, or as a temporary measure whilst arrangements for long-term feeding arrangements are being made.

Enteral nutrition (nasal tube and jejunostomy)

The preferred route for introducing nutrition into the body is directly through the gastrointestinal tract (enteral nutrition). This ensures that the intestines are kept active, and outcomes are better when this route is used. Enteral nutrition is commonly provided using a nasal tube or a surgical jejunostomy.

A nasal tube (sometimes referred to as a naso-gastric/NG or naso-jejunal/NJ tube) is a very slim tube which is placed up the nose, down the throat, and either into or just past the stomach (or pouch) into the small intestine. These tubes can be placed using a gastroscope (camera) or using X-rays to guide the procedure. Nasal tubes are usually used as a short-term option as they can irritate the throat and sometimes fall out.

A surgical jejunostomy is a tube which is introduced through the skin and directly into the first part of the small intestine (called the jejunum). It is placed by a surgeon whilst under a general anaesthetic and is often undertaken using a laparoscopic (keyhole) approach. A jejunostomy is usually a longer-term option to support nutrition and may be offered in scenarios where healing may take a long time (from a leak for example), or whilst further tests and treatments are being planned.

Summary

In summary, revision surgery is a complex area that needs careful work-up and investigation by an experienced team who have taken the time to identify the specific problems that need addressing. Quite often, more surgery is not the solution to most problems which may arise following bariatric surgery. However, in those cases where it *is* deemed appropriate, revision surgery is safe and can be effective.

Chapter 6: Preparing for surgery

What is covered in this chapter?

- Initial consultation and booking surgery.
- Pre-operative assessment.
- Patient responsibilities before surgery.

Introduction

As ever, preparation for the big day is key and will give you the best chance of recovering well and getting the best results in the long term. This section will cover the process which takes place ahead of surgery from your initial consultation up to the day of admission for your procedure. Having a clear understanding of what to expect in the run up, will for most people, alleviate many of the anxieties and uncertainties associated with the process.

The initial consultation

Initial consultations are an opportunity for you to gain a better understanding of medical treatments for weight loss and begin building a relationship with your surgeon. Nowadays, initial consultations can be arranged to take place face to face, via video call or over the telephone giving you the flexibility to work around a busy schedule. In the UK, appointments for privately self-funded care can be arranged directly by contacting a surgeon's practice or through the hospital in which they work.

During the initial appointment, you will have the opportunity to discuss any aspects of your care and have all your questions answered. My advice is to prepare a list of questions for the surgeon, including questions about the different procedures, possible complications and what aftercare is included. In my practice, you will be asked to complete a comprehensive online medical questionnaire to support this process, and this will be reviewed during your consultation. We will then discuss the different options available to you and ensure that you are offered choices tailored to your set of unique circumstances. Sometimes, follow-up appointments are required before proceeding with surgery.

Information needed prior to your consultation

If you have significant medical conditions, it is always useful to have a copy of correspondence or letters from your hospital specialists which can speed up the decision-making process. For example, if you are diabetic, it is important to understand how well controlled your blood sugars are as this can impact on recovery and complication rates. Sometimes it is necessary to postpone surgery if blood sugar control is poor. Another common example relates to patients who have previous heart conditions. If you have had recent investigations such as an echocardiogram or a 24-hour heart tracing, a report or formal correspondence which confirms these results is necessary before surgery can proceed.

Decision-making and any recommendations made during your consultation process are based largely on the information you provide about your health. Whilst most surgical practices will normally go to significant lengths to make sure that all the necessary information is available ahead of surgery, this will only be possible through your active engagement with the process. On rare occasions where incomplete or inaccurate information is provided, this may result in the postponement or cancellation of surgery if it is deemed, for example, that you do not fulfil the eligibility criteria or that further information and investigations are required. In my practice, we will always ask you for consent to contact your GP and ensure that your medical records are kept complete and up to date.

Booking and Timing of Surgery

Once you have had an opportunity to reflect on the outcome of your consultation and wish or able to proceed, the next step is to contact the team to arrange a date for surgery. If you are paying for your procedure (or if you have medical insurance which covers weight loss treatments) you will usually have more influence on when this can take place. Deciding on when to have your procedure should be a carefully considered choice. Not only should you be physically and psychologically prepared, but you should also carefully consider the impacts on work and whether you will have the necessary support at that time. If you have been referred for surgery through a public healthcare system (such as the UK's National Health Service – NHS), the timing of surgery may be influenced by other factors such as waiting list times (which will be covered below).

There may be other factors to think about as well. I often speak to women who have recently given birth and are concerned about the impact of surgery on breastfeeding. Whilst current guidelines suggest that breastfeeding after anaesthetic is usually safe (as soon as mother is alert and able to), you should also be mindful that with the significantly reduced oral intake after surgery, it is unlikely that the same volume of breast milk will continue.

If you have undergone surgery recently or experienced a major life event, you will need to make sure that you have recovered both physically and mentally. This is so you can focus on the post-operative recovery and give yourself the best chance of maximising results in the long-term. We will talk about this in greater detail later.

The steps in booking your procedure may vary between practices. In my practice, you would call the team and discuss available surgery dates. Once this has been agreed, a booking form is submitted to the hospital, which then triggers several further appointments with pre-operative assessment, the bariatric nurses, and dietitians. Where necessary, an appointment with a psychologist or psychotherapist may also be arranged.

NHS Pathways

For patients undergoing bariatric surgery through the NHS, the process leading up to surgery is very different and varies significantly between regions. If you fulfil the eligibility criteria for bariatric surgery, a referral to a weight management programme can be made through your GP. In exceptional circumstances, there may be fast-track referral pathways available in cases where urgent weight loss is required to treat other life-threatening conditions such as cancer, for example. Once you have completed a period in weight management (this can vary from 6 to 12 months, or more), you will be referred to the surgical team to be considered for surgery. This is a grossly simplistic view of the NHS referral pathway. In reality, the timelines for this process can take years – particularly for routine referrals – which is why many people opt to privately fund weight loss surgery.

Pre-operative assessment

All patients in my practice must undergo a comprehensive pre-operative assessment which aims to make sure that surgery can be carried out safely. This includes physical, nutritional and psychological assessments, medical background checks (including a review of current medications), swabs, and an ECG heart tracing. You will also undergo several bloods tests which aim to explore all major body systems (including liver and kidney function), rule out any pre-existing micronutrient deficiencies (such as Vitamin D and iron deficiencies) and ensure that blood sugar levels are well controlled. On rare occasions, new, previously undiagnosed medical conditions (such as diabetes) are discovered, or concerns regarding psychological preparedness for surgery are raised. These may require additional investigation and treatment that could result in the postponement of surgery. Similarly, if additional psychological assessment or support is required ahead of surgery, this will be arranged.

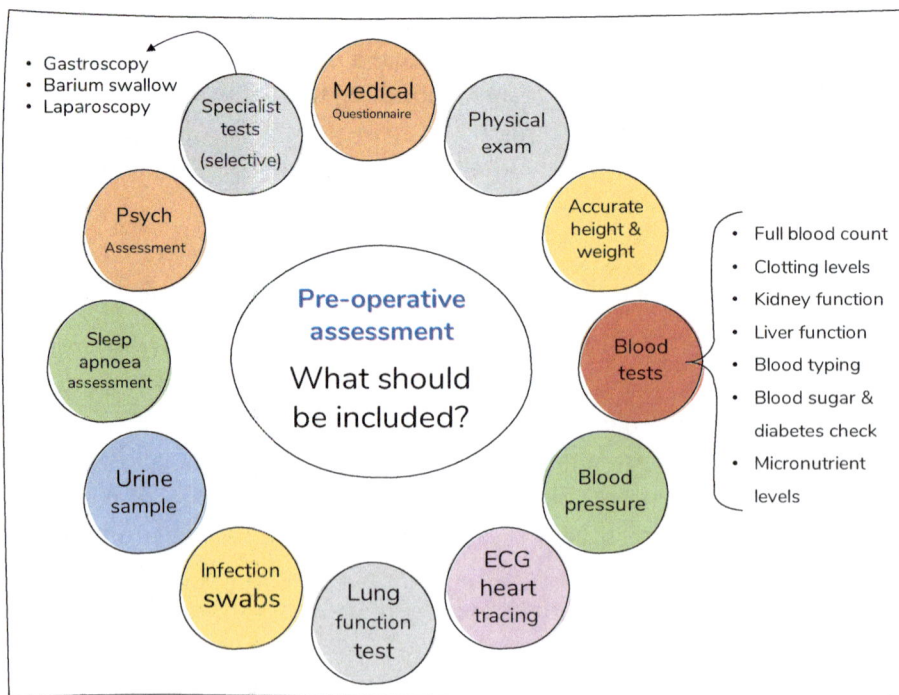

You will also have a blood sample taken to check your blood type in the rare case that you need a blood transfusion after surgery. If you have an objection to receiving blood products, please highlight these in advance so that alternative arrangements can be made.

Whilst not routinely performed in the UK, gastroscopy (also known as endoscopy or a camera test) of your oesophagus and stomach can be useful in identifying conditions for which you do not have symptoms. In some cases, it may also be necessary to undertake an X-ray test called a barium swallow of your oesophagus and stomach. This may help your surgical team better plan the most appropriate surgery and treatments for you.

Obstructive Sleep Apnoea

As we have previously covered, obstructive sleep apnoea (OSA) is a common sleep disorder characterized by pauses in breathing or shallow breaths during sleep. It occurs when the muscles in the back of the throat fail to keep the airway open during sleep, despite the effort to breathe. As a result, the airway becomes partially or completely blocked. These pauses can last for a few seconds to several minutes and can occur multiple times throughout the night, disrupting the quality of sleep and leading to symptoms such as loud snoring, gasping or choking during sleep, and excessive daytime sleepiness.

OSA can affect individuals of any age, but it is more common in those who are overweight, have a family history of the condition, or have certain anatomical features that narrow the airway, such as a large tongue, tonsils, or a small jaw. Other risk factors include smoking, alcohol use, and certain medications.

Untreated OSA can lead to a variety of health problems, including high blood pressure, stroke, heart disease, diabetes, depression, and cognitive impairment. All patients are screened for sleep apnoea during their pre-operative assessment process. If left untreated, OSA can be dangerous after surgery because the medications used during anaesthesia can make the muscles in the throat and tongue relax even more than they would during sleep, leading to a greater risk of airway obstruction and breathing difficulties.

During your pre-operative assessment, your risk of underlying OSA will be assessed. If your risk is high, it is likely you will need to undergo formal sleep studies to confirm the diagnosis. Once confirmed, most people will need to be issued with a CPAP machine to improve breathing during sleep. Once you are established on this, surgery can be safely undertaken, and most hospitals will be happy to care for you in a normal ward. An alternative approach would be to nurse you in a high dependency unit (HDU) post-operatively which would normally result in additional costs. If you are already established on CPAP, it is important to bring this with you to the hospital so that it can be used during your stay whilst you sleep.

Patient responsibilities

Losing weight before surgery

Generally, there is no requirement to lose a specific amount of weight before surgery. However, in some cases, it may be necessary to set a weight loss goal before surgery to ensure that the procedure can be carried out safely. This is especially the case if your BMI is greater than 60 kg/m^2. Please make sure you clarify this with your surgical team. Any weight that is lost before surgery is weight that will be kept off in the longer term so there are additional benefits to losing weight pre-operatively.

The liver reducing diet (LRD)

The liver lies directly over the stomach, which needs to be accessed safely during surgery. We ask patients to strictly adhere to a liver reducing diet (LRD) to shrink the liver and allow it to be gently moved aside more easily. The details of this diet and how long you should adhere to it will be provided to you ahead of surgery. There are usually three types of LRD which can be followed. These include a 'milk and yoghurt diet', 'fluid-based meal replacement' or 'food-based diet'. Each of these aims to limit the calorie intake to approximately 800kcal a day primarily by reducing carbohydrate and fat consumption. Whilst protein rich foods are encouraged, it is usual to see protein intake reduce as well in an attempt to meet the calorie target.

If the LRD is not adhered to, there is a risk that surgery becomes more technically challenging and that it cannot be completed as planned. Sometimes this means that surgery is abandoned altogether. As this will not be known until during the time of surgery, you may be liable for any costs incurred, including a portion of the hospital, surgeon, and anaesthetic fees.

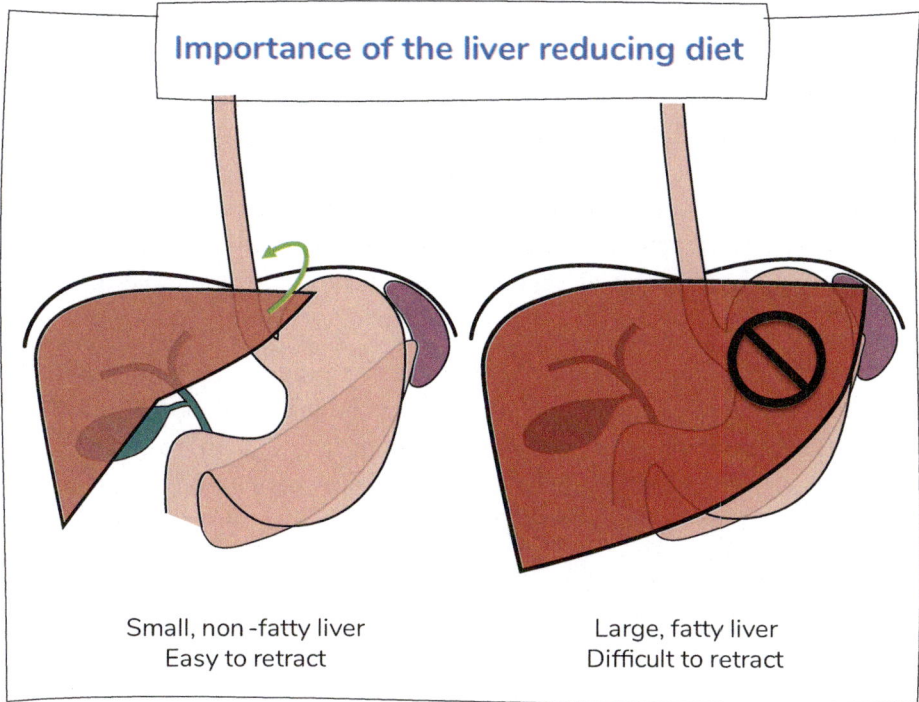

Importance of the liver reducing diet

Small, non-fatty liver
Easy to retract

Large, fatty liver
Difficult to retract

Do I need to let my doctor know I am having surgery?

I strongly advise you to let your GP or primary care physician know about any intentions to pursue weight loss surgery. In the UK, your GP practice will play an important role in prescribing medications and undertaking blood tests after your procedure. Giving them prior notice of your intention is good practice and gives us an opportunity to iron out any concerns they may have about your follow up care.

If you suffer from conditions that are under the care of specialist medial teams or that require medications, it may be necessary to inform them prior to surgery. Pre-existing conditions may impact on the type and timing of the procedure you can have. Weight loss surgery can also impact on how medications are absorbed by the body. If this is the case, my practice is to contact the medical team or GP for further assistance. It is therefore useful for you to have the names and contact details of relevant medical teams ahead of your initial consultation.

Smoking & Nicotine Use

If you use nicotine products (including cigarettes, vape and tobacco packets) you will be required to stop before surgery and commit to not starting again in the future. In my practice, I ask people to smoking at least 6 weeks before their procedure, although this may be shorter or longer depending on the surgeon's preference. In addition to other health risks, nicotine use significantly increases the risks of serious complications around the time of surgery, such as poor healing, and leaks from staple lines and surgical joins.

Smoking also increases your chance of developing stomach inflammation and ulcers in the future. A history of smoking and the likelihood of restarting may influence the type of recommendations made with respect to the procedures offered. For example, a gastric bypass may be a less favourable option if you have been a long-term smoker due to the risks of chronic stomach ulceration.

Alcohol Intake

During your consultation, we will also discuss your alcohol intake. For some people, alcohol can be a daily feature in their lives. After surgery, we recommend you avoid alcohol for at least 6 months to prioritise more nutrient dense food and drink. If you drink heavily, you may unknowingly be reliant on alcohol, and this can jeopardise your recovery and long-term results. Therefore, at the very least, I will ask patients to reduce their alcohol intake to below the recommended weekly limits in the run up to their surgery. If needed, your surgery may need to be postponed so that that this can be achieved safely.

Optimising Your Health

Most patients who I speak to will have at least one or more weight-related medical conditions. We have already talked about the importance of optimising diabetes control and identifying undiagnosed conditions such as sleep apnoea before surgery. But there are many other conditions that may need to be optimised so surgery can take place safely. These include problems related to the heart and lungs and of course issues related to mental health. If you have these conditions, it may be necessary to postpone surgery until we are happy that your procedure can be undertaken safely.

Medication management

We generally ask you to continue most medications up to the day of surgery. These will be reviewed by the pharmacist and bariatric nurse ahead in the run up to your operation and should be brought into the hospital with you. These include:

- Blood pressure tablets.
- Medications for diabetes – although these may need to be adjusted to avoid low blood sugars on the day of surgery.
- Thyroxine for those who have underactive thyroid.
- Medications for asthma such as inhalers.
- Tablets for acid reflux.

However, there are certain medications which will ask you to stop in the lead up to surgery such as:

- Blood thinning medications like warfarin, aspirin, clopidogrel and apixaban which can increase the risk of bleeding at the time of surgery.
- Some anti-inflammatory medications like Naproxen which can increase the risks of bleeding.
- Biologic medications such as those used with rheumatoid arthritis which can increase problems with healing.
- Oestrogen hormone-based medications such as HRT and the combined contraceptive pill approximately 4-weeks before surgery as they can increase the risk of blood clots.

A clear management plan for the use of these medications will be provided to so you know what to do well ahead of surgery. On the day of surgery, the anaesthetist will review your medications with you to determine which regular medications you should omit.

Hormonal Medication Management

For women undergoing bariatric surgery, the contraceptive pill and HRT are commonly used to control a wide range of symptoms which severely affect quality of life. Largely, these can be continued safely around the time surgery. However, patients should be aware that certain types of the oral contraceptive pill – in particular the combined pill - and HRT tablets which contain oestrogen can increase the chances of developing blood clots in the leg. These blood clots can potentially travel to the lung to cause pulmonary embolism, which in some rare cases can be life-threatening.

Whilst a strict protocol after surgery ensures that everyone is given blood thinning medication to reduce this risk, patients are given the choice to discontinue the pill and HRT if they wish for about 1 month before surgery. The progesterone only mini-pill and HRT patches (and other formulas including gels) are safe to continue.

Following surgery, the absorption of some medications, including the oral contraceptive pill can be altered. The use of alternative methods of contraception such as implants, barrier methods or the intra-uterine device are therefore advised.

Weight Loss Medication

For several reasons, patients may be taking medications for weight loss in the run up to surgery. These include GLP-1 injectable medications such as semaglutide and liraglutide. I am often asked whether these are safe to continue in the run up to surgery. Whilst these are largely safe, there is some evidence which suggests that they can affect the way in which the stomach works and increase the risk of nausea and vomiting in the post-operative period. It is important to discuss this with your surgeon.

Preparing for Life after surgery

Education and knowledge building

In addition to reading material and other resources such as this book, you will receive tailored information and advice regarding life after surgery from the wider team including bariatric nurses, dietitians, and if necessary, psychologists and pharmacists. This should happen before your operation, to give you an opportunity to prepare mentally, have realistic expectations, and put into place the necessary measures to give you the best chance of long-term success.

Lifestyle changes & Support systems

As we have previously discussed, obesity develops due to a complex combination of different reasons. In the run up to surgery it is important to understand your own factors which contributed to obesity so that robust plans can be put into place to address and avoid these as best as possible in the future. This will give you the best chance of controlling your weight and any related medical conditions in the long-term.

Most people begin to make nutritional changes in preparation for life after surgery. This includes cutting out sugars, fizzy drinks and alcohol and focussing on more nutrient dense options which are high in proteins, healthy fats, and fibre. Eating at regular intervals will help you get into good habits as will achieving a daily fluid target of around 2 litres in the run up to surgery, particularly if this is something you are not accustomed to. Nutritional tips after surgery are covered in greater detail later, but in principle can be adopted before surgery in preparation for life after surgery.

Patients undergoing bariatric surgery also benefit from having a strong support system in place, including family, friends, and support groups. You should work with your aftercare team and GP practice to identify resources that can help them succeed before and after surgery. We will discuss the important topic of support in greater detail elsewhere.

Chapter 7: What to expect in hospital

What is covered in this chapter?

- What happens before surgery.
- What happens during your operation.
- Recovering in hospital.

Introduction

In this section we will discuss what to expect during your stay in hospital including people you will meet, the step-by-step process of what happens in the run up to your procedure and other common questions I am asked about recovery in hospital. Each surgical practice is set up slightly differently, and therefore local practices may vary. The overview presented here reflects my own practice and will serve as a good indicator with respect to what you can expect.

Arriving at the Hospital

The time allocated for arrival to the hospital largely depends on the time the operating lists begin. If the operating list starts in the morning or lasts all day, you will be asked to attend the hospital around 7am on the day of your surgery. After being shown to your room and completing some initial checks, and women will be asked to provide a urine sample for a pregnancy test. You will meet several members of the team including myself, the anaesthetist, and the surgical assistant. Each will go through a list of questions, discuss their contribution to your care and reiterate the benefits and risks associated with the planned procedure. The anaesthetist will also review any regular medications and decide which of these can be taken that day. You will have the opportunity to ask any further questions and confirm that you still wish to proceed with your procedure by signing a consent form.

Clothing and other preparations

After your initial checks have been completed, you will be asked to change into a surgical gown and put on some stockings (known as TED - thrombo-embolic deterrent - stockings) which improve the blood circulation in your legs and reduce the risk of blood clots. In my practice, I also give a dose of a blood thinning injection to reduce this risk further before surgery takes place. You will also be given some medications which aim to reduce acid reflux and nausea.

The hospital may ask you to remove piercings and nail polish (or acrylic nails) before your surgery so please make sure to check about this beforehand. If you have hair extensions which contain metal clips, it is important to let the team know as this may cause a risk of burns during surgery. Finally, people prioritise their concerns differently. If you have any questions which have not been answered in this section, my advice is to ask your team either ahead of time, or on the day or surgery.

Time of surgery

Operating lists can last all day and there are usually several patients undergoing surgery. The order of the operating list depends on many factors including the complexity of the cases taking place that day, with more complex patients and cases such as those undergoing revision surgery or who are diabetic being prioritised ahead of others.

Whilst the order of the cases is planned well in advance, a final short planning meeting takes place in the morning and the final list order is confirmed. Following this, you will be given an approximate time to expect when your surgery will take place. I usually encourage you to bring something to occupy your time (such as a book or electronic device), particularly if your surgery is planned for the afternoon or in case there are any unexpected delays.

Eating & drinking before surgery

During your pre-operative assessment, you will be given details about when to stop eating and drinking prior to admission to hospital. Usually, I ask patients to stop eating at midnight before surgery which allows the stomach to be completely empty by the time of surgery. After this time, you will be allowed to drink clear water up until 6am. If you are not having surgery right at the start of the day, you will be encouraged to continue drinking water. Remaining well hydrated during the day improves the patient experience and reduces the severity of post-operative nausea. Fluid policies vary from practice to practice – some may ask you to drink up to 2 hours before your procedure, but others may allow you to drink water more frequently, or even take some black tea or coffee.

The anaesthetic

Before you leave your room, the nursing staff will undertake an additional check to ensure all your personal details are correct. A member of staff will walk with you from your room to the operating theatre complex and take you into the anaesthetic room or directly into the operating theatre where you will be taken through another brief checklist.

Following this, the team will prepare you for the general anaesthetic which includes placing a small cannula (also known as an intravenous line) in the back of your hand. This may have already been done by a member of staff whilst you were on the ward. You will be asked to hold an oxygen mask to your face as the anaesthetic takes effect. As soon as you are asleep, the anaesthetist will place a tube down into the airway to support your breathing during the procedure and continue to monitor you closely throughout the procedure.

I am often asked about the safety of anaesthesia in the context of obesity. You should be reassured that anaesthesia is very safe. In my practice I only work with a very small number of anaesthetists with a specialist interest in bariatric anaesthesia, which further reduces the small associated risks.

Length of procedure

The length of procedure can vary depending on many factors, the most important being the type of procedure or surgery you are undergoing:

- The band and sleeve gastrectomy may take around 30-60 minutes
- The mini gastric bypass between 45-90 minutes and
- The full gastric bypass around an hour to two hours

Of course, revision surgery will usually prolong the procedure time, as will having a very large liver – which is partly why we ask you to stick to a liver reducing diet in the run up to surgery. Other reasons why surgery may take longer, include the presence of scar tissue from previous surgery or unexpected findings that need attention such as a hiatus hernia.

Patients also spend about 15 to 20 minutes in the theatre complex before surgery undergoing additional checks and being put to sleep. Immediately after surgery, the anaesthetic is reversed after which you spend between 30 and 60 minutes recovering from anaesthesia in the theatre complex. The recovery nurses will ensure that any symptoms of discomfort or nausea are well-controlled and that the effects of the anaesthetic have largely worn off before you are taken back to your room. In summary you can expect to be away from your room for at least 2 hours regardless of which procedure you are having.

Unexpected findings during surgery

At the start of surgery, I will normally look at the visible internal organs to ensure that no undiagnosed problems are present. Depending on the findings, I will assess whether it is safe to proceed with surgery as planned. Sometimes it is necessary and safer to postpone bariatric surgery until further tests and investigations have been carried out.

Significant steps are taken to minimise the risk of not being able to proceed with your surgery as planned. Whilst this is exceptionally rare, findings at surgery can be unpredictable and your safety is the single most important priority. Reasons that may result in either a change to the planned procedure or completely abandoning surgery include:

- A large liver (due to not strictly adhering to the liver shrinking diet)
- Severe adhesions or scarring (such as those from previous surgery or medical conditions such as endometriosis)
- Technical factors that would make the procedure unsafe to undertake (for example in the case of a bypass if we were not safely able to join the small bowel to the stomach pouch).
- Other unexpected findings that require further investigations
- Or a complication from surgery

Thankfully the chance of unexpected findings which result in not being able to perform any type of weight loss surgery is very rare.

Hiatus hernia

A hiatus hernia occurs when part of the stomach protrudes through the diaphragm (the thin sheet of muscle that separates the chest and abdominal cavities).

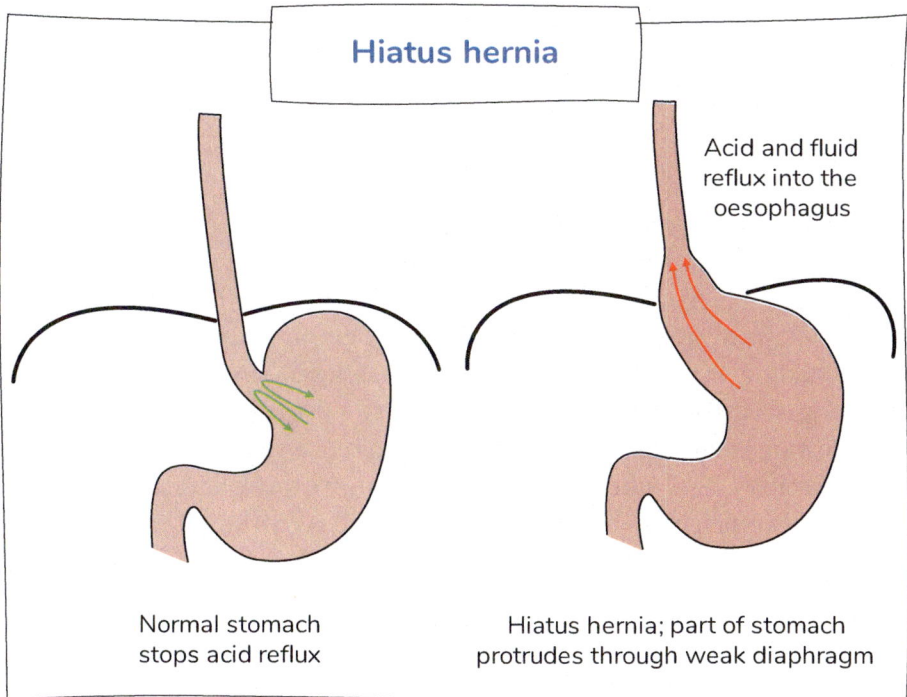

Hiatus hernia

Acid and fluid reflux into the oesophagus

Normal stomach stops acid reflux

Hiatus hernia; part of stomach protrudes through weak diaphragm

It is not uncommon for a previously undiagnosed hiatus hernia to be found during weight loss surgery. This usually requires repair to reduce the risk of future problems such as difficulty swallowing, heartburn and reflux symptoms which can significantly impact on quality of life.

The risks of repairing a hiatus hernia are small. In addition to the risks associated with your surgery, these include failure to improve any existing heartburn or reflux-related symptoms, recurrence of symptoms in the future, Dumping syndrome (which we will talk about later), difficulty swallowing or the sensation of food sticking in the oesophagus. As with any other unexpected finding, your surgeon will need to assess whether it is safe to proceed with the proposed bariatric surgery, especially if the hernia is very large.

Combined Surgeries

Sometimes patients undergoing weight loss surgery have other pre-existing conditions such as symptomatic gallstones or hernias (including an umbilical or hiatus hernia) that require operations to treat. In some cases, it may be possible to undertake this additional procedure at the same time of bariatric surgery. However, your surgeon's preference may be to focus solely on your weight loss procedure and leave these other conditions to be treated another time.

As we have discussed above, a known (or previously undiagnosed) hiatus hernia would usually need to be repaired at the same time of bariatric surgery as it can significantly impact on outcomes and recovery. With respect to gallbladder surgery, some surgeons may offer to remove this at the same time to save you from an additional general anaesthetic and further recovery time. You should be aware however that additional procedures may prolong your recovery from weight loss surgery, may also increase the risk of complications and likely attract an additional cost. In the case of umbilical (naval) hernias, it may be more appropriate to fix these at a later date once you have lost weight, to reduce the risk of these recurring.

Waking up from surgery

As soon as your operation has been completed, you are carefully transferred from the operating table and back into your bed. At this point, the anaesthetic team will 'reverse' the anaesthetic and wake you up. This process normally happens in the operating theatre itself, but sometimes may happen in a facility immediately next to the operating theatre called the 'recovery area'. You will be taken to the recovery area in your bed where you will be cared for by specially trained staff who ensure that you are progressing well and that any pain, discomfort, and nausea is well controlled.

Most people will be groggy after their anaesthetic and this feeling will continue for a few hours. After around 20 to 30 minutes in the recovery area, you will be transferred in your bed back up to the ward to continue your recovery.

What scars will I have after surgery?

With the sleeve gastrectomy, gastric bypass and gastric band, you will have four or five small keyhole incisions which are typically between 5mm and 15mm long. There are typically two on either side of the abdomen and then three on the front of the abdomen.

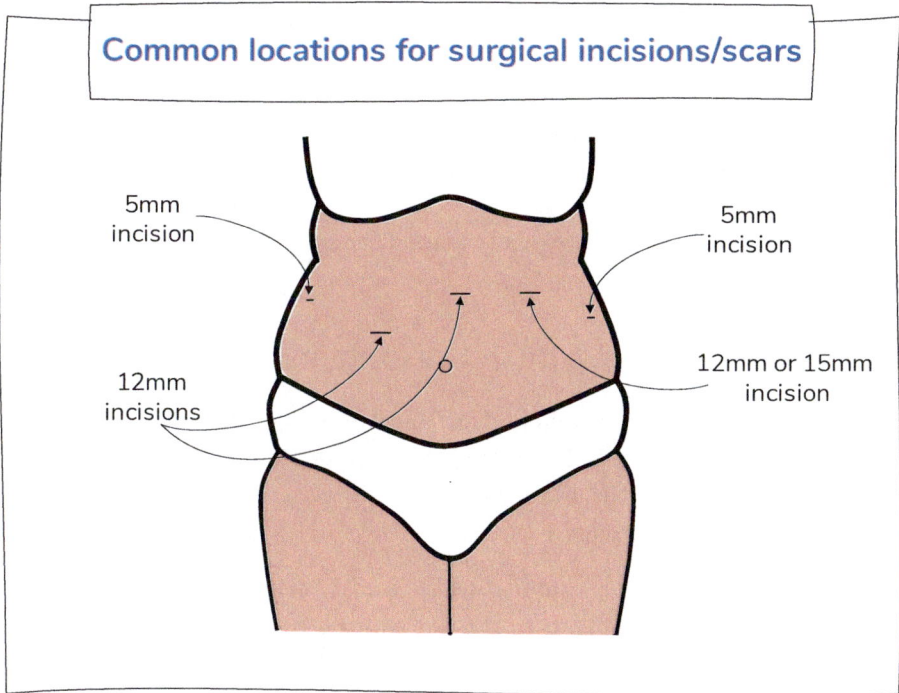

Common locations for surgical incisions/scars

5mm incision

5mm incision

12mm incisions

12mm or 15mm incision

In my practice, the wounds are closed using a combination of dissolvable sutures and skin glue ensuring you have the best chance of healing neatly. The incisions will be waterproof within 24 hours, allowing you to have a shower. I encourage patients to pat their wounds dry to stop them accidently rubbing off the skin glue, which will naturally fall off by 2 weeks after surgery. In some cases, patients may develop an allergic reaction to skin glue, although the risk of this is rare.

If you have had previous laparoscopic (keyhole) surgery (to remove your gallbladder or previous weight loss surgery for example) it is often possible to use at least some of the previous incisions. Of course, this may not always be possible, but if this is an important consideration for you, please make sure you bring this point up with your surgeon.

In extraordinarily rare cases, laparoscopic surgery cannot be undertaken safely, and a large open incision to the abdomen is needed. This may be due to a complication which requires immediate and urgent treatment. Complications aside, if surgery cannot be safely undertaken using a laparoscopic approach (perhaps due to severe adhesions or scarring), I would rather abandon the operation than convert to a large open incision.

I often get asked about wound drains. My practice is not to need these routinely, whilst other surgeons may do so. Please make sure you speak to your surgeon about this beforehand. Similarly, if you have skin tattoos, it is worthwhile to speak to your surgeon about the placement of the incisions. Quite often these can be strategically placed to reduce the risk of interrupting tattoos.

How visible will scars be in the long-term?

By the time the glue has flaked off between one and two weeks after surgery, your wounds will be completely healed. Quite often it can take between 6-12 months for the scars to disappears. The visibility of scars depends on several factors:

- Nutritional status: Adequate nutrition is crucial for proper wound healing after bariatric surgery. Ensuring a balanced and nutrient-dense diet which allows sufficient protein, vitamins, and minerals will give you the best chance of good healing.
- Obesity-related health conditions: Patients with obesity-related health conditions, such as type 2 diabetes, may experience slower wound healing after bariatric surgery. Close monitoring of blood glucose levels can help minimize this risk.
- Skin type: Darker skin types may result in more pigmented or overgrowth of scarring (called hypertrophic scars) which can be challenging to treat.
- Incision location and size: The location and size of the incision can affect how well it heals. Smaller incisions tend to heal faster than larger incisions. Incisions that are made in areas with more movement, such as the abdomen, may require longer healing times.

- Wound care: Proper wound care is crucial for promoting healing after bariatric surgery. Incisions should largely be kept clean and dry, and any signs of infection, such as redness, swelling, or leakage should be reported early.
- Smoking and alcohol use: Smoking and alcohol use can interfere with the body's healing processes and increase the risk of complications after surgery. Patients should avoid smoking and limit alcohol consumption in the weeks before and after surgery.
- Follow-up care: Regular follow-up appointments with the healthcare provider can help identify any potential issues with the incisions and ensure that healing is progressing as expected.

What will I be expected to do when I return to the ward?

Many practices, including my own, have developed strict protocols to ensure that your post-operative course is as predictable as possible. These protocols aim to streamline your recovery by removing variation, and work partly by prompting medical, nursing staff and patients to undertake particular tasks and achieve certain goals during recovery. For example, when you return to the ward, the nursing staff will regularly take your blood pressure, heart rate, and check on your oxygen levels.

On the day of surgery, you will be asked to sip water and encouraged to mobilise to and from the toilet with help from the nurses and healthcare assistants. Later in the day, you will be encouraged to walk the length of the ward corridor as well. Achieving these milestones help us witness progress so that we can work towards appropriate and safe discharge, usually the following day.

Managing pain, nausea and vomiting

The amount of pain and discomfort that people feel after surgery varies. Some people will have very little pain or discomfort, whilst most will have some symptoms. This is due to a combination of the incisions and the carbon dioxide gas that we use to be able to perform the surgery (commonly referred to as 'gas or wind pain'). Gas pain is often felt at the top of the abdomen and sometimes in the shoulders. This is because nerves connect the diaphragm to the shoulders; irritation of the diaphragm can therefore be referred to and felt in the shoulder.

Expectations after bariatric surgery

Day of surgery	Day after surgery
Sipping 30-60mls of water per hour	Sipping 100mls of fluids per hour
Dressed in own clothes	Dressed in own clothes
Mobilising to the toilet	Mobilising unassisted
Walk up and down the ward	Prepare for discharge

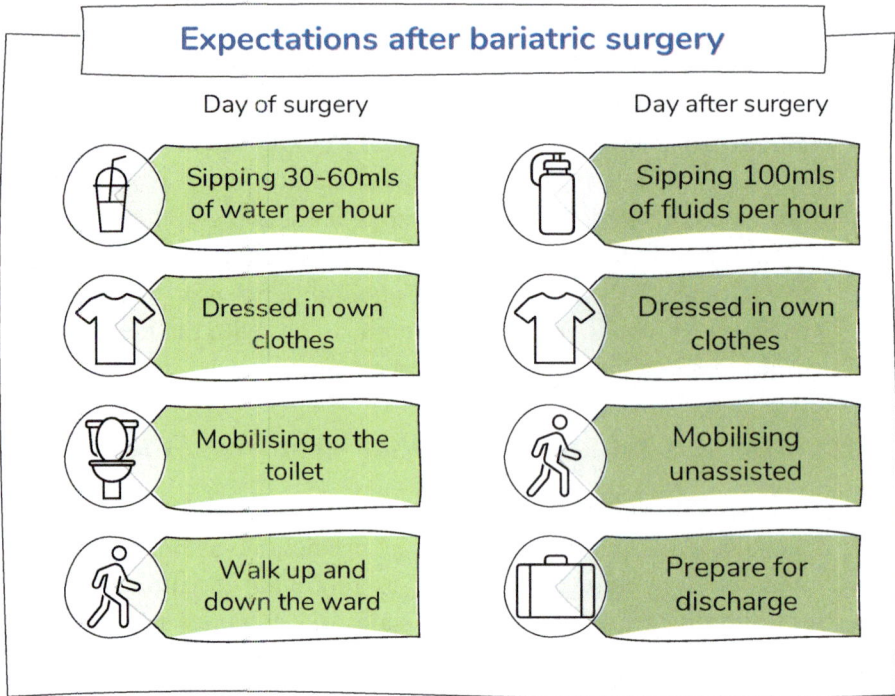

One of the reasons we encourage you to remain mobile after surgery is that it significantly can relieve abdominal discomfort, alongside using other approaches such as drinking peppermint tea. Sometimes patients can also have pain on swallowing fluid in the days after their procedure, which is entirely normal and a reflection of the inflammation and swelling from your surgery.

The team can take additional steps to minimise pain by removing as much gas as possible at the end of the surgery and using local anaesthetic to the wounds. We also make sure that pain relief is given before, during and after surgery to help your recovery. Some people also struggle with nausea and vomiting in the first few days after their surgery, which is why we make sure that patients have a comprehensive review by our pharmacists and are given several medications to use following discharge. In the first 24 hours after surgery, it is common for vomiting to be blood-stained. This is often self-limiting and does not require any treatment or intervention.

Length of stay in Hospital

The amount of time that you remain in hospital depends on several factors including the type of procedure you are undergoing.

- If you are having a gastric balloon or a gastric band, you will most likely be able to go home on the same day of your procedure.
- If you are having a sleeve, bypass, or some type of revision surgery, you will likely be in hospital for no more one- or two-days following surgery.
- Sometimes it is necessary to stay in longer to ensure that you are drinking enough, and that symptoms of discomfort and nausea are well controlled.

Discharge from hospital

As part of the enhanced recovery protocol, there are strict guidelines that will determine whether you safe to be discharged from hospital. This includes ensuring that you are mobile and self-caring (such as be able to use the bathroom), pain and nausea symptoms are well controlled, and that you are tolerating an adequate volume of fluid (usually in the region of around 100 ml every hour). If these criteria are not met, then your stay in hospital is extended until you are safe to leave.

Prior to discharge, you will be reviewed by members of the surgical, nursing and aftercare team and be given the opportunity to ask further questions. The specialist pharmacist will also review any regular medications you take to ensure that large tablets that cannot be crushed or dissolved are converted to liquid form. In addition, you will be given several medications to take at home including:

- Pain killers.
- Anti-sickness medication.
- Medication to reduce stomach acid production.
- And injections for at least one week to thin the blood and reduce the risk of developing blood clots. This course may be extended if you have a previous history of blood clots, medical conditions that increase your risks, a BMI of over 60 or significant problems with mobilising.

Fit notes (also known as 'sick' notes)

Many people worry about whether they can take sick leave for bariatric surgery and are anxious about work-colleagues finding out about their procedure. As we have discussed before, bariatric surgery is <u>not</u> cosmetic surgery and focuses on improving health. It should be considered no different from other types of elective surgery such as a joint replacement.

Fit notes are normally available from the ward on request and are completed to state that you have undergone 'surgery' without disclosing the type of procedure you have undergone. For most people, I provide a two-week fit note for you to present to work. If you require longer, or a phased return due to the nature of your work, this can either be arranged in advance or after discharge by contacting your GP.

Travelling home

On discharge, you will need to arrange to be picked up from the hospital and accompanied home. You should also ensure that you have the support of family or friends in the first week whilst you recover from your procedure. If you live a significant distance away from the hospital, I always recommend that you book a stay at a local hotel for the first few nights so that you can present back at the hospital promptly should a problem arise.

Whilst travelling home, make sure that you can take a regular break. Remember to continue with fluids to remain hydrated, and stop at least every hour if travelling by car to stretch your legs to reduce the risk of developing blood clots.

Communication and Advice for your GP

Communication between your surgical team and primary care doctor is key for several reasons. At the very least, GPs will be responsible for managing regular medications that you already take, and an understanding of how bariatric surgery may affect this is necessary. This is especially the case for diabetes and blood pressure medication.

Some GPs will also be responsible for the prescription of nutritional supplementation and regular blood-testing post-operatively. In my practice, a discharge document which includes key recommendations for follow-up and medicine management is provided to your GP. This will also provide information should the doctor wish to contact the surgical team for any reason.

What if my GP won't provide support for me after surgery?

Care for bariatric surgery undertaken by the NHS will be fully supported by your GP and will take place in collaboration with the NHS hospital. What this support looks like will vary between regions. With respect to privately funded surgery, most GPs in the UK will provide support in the form of prescriptions and blood tests, particularly if this comes at the request of a surgical team who provide clear guidance on what that entails. More specialised follow up will be provided by your aftercare team. What that includes should be clear to both you and your GP so that there is no ambiguity.

In the rarer cases where GPs are unable to support you following surgery, it is important to understand the reasons why. Sometimes this is because they do not feel it is within their scope of expertise, at which point a more collaborative approach with the aftercare team may be required. Very rarely, patients are told by GPs that they have been directed by governing authorities not to support privately funded bariatric surgery. In these rare cases, you are still able to undergo surgery, but will need to pay privately for supplementation and blood tests. This is a lifelong financial cost that you will need to consider ahead of surgery. There are now a growing number of private GPs with an interest in weight management who are able to oversee this aspect of your care.

Chapter 8: Recovering from surgery

What is covered in this chapter?

- Recommendations during recovery.
- Challenges in the post-operative period.
- How to spot complications.

Introduction

We now move onto the period of recovery after surgery which typically involves several phases. This *can* vary depending on several factors, including the type of procedure performed and the individual patient's condition. These phases can be split into:

- Early postoperative recovery for the first two weeks after surgery.
- A period of adapting to your post-surgery life which usually lasts around 3 months.
- A late phase which focuses on maximising weight loss.
- Maintenance phase which focuses on sustaining weight loss and maximising health and quality of life in the long-term.

This chapter focuses on physical recovery during the first few months after discharge from hospital.

Early post-operative phase

For those who have undergone surgery, most people will be self-caring immediately after discharge and encouraged to remain mobile and well hydrated. This will speed up recovery and reduce the risk of complications such as blood clots. You can expect to see gradual improvements in discomfort and mobility during the first week. By the end of the second week most people will have completed their physical recovery and should not have any significant pain or limitations in their mobility.

Additional support from others

Each person's circumstances and requirements are unique. However, most people will need some additional support from family and friends in the first few days. This is particularly important if you have dependents such as children that have needs such as pick-ups and drop offs to school. Remember, if at any point you feel overwhelmed or uncertain, you should be able to contact your aftercare team for guidance.

Resuming daily activities

Because surgery is undertaken using a keyhole or laparoscopic approach, most people are able resume their normal day to day activities as soon as they feel up to it. However, I would usually advise you not to drive before two weeks following surgery. In UK law, there is no predefined period before which you can start driving after surgery. You will need to make that assessment yourself by making sure that you are in full control of the vehicle and can perform an emergency stop. Most insurance companies will stipulate that your ability to drive must not be impaired to be covered by your policy.

Returning to work

The time it takes to get back to work depends on the nature of your work. For most people, they can resume work by the time their physical recovery is complete at around 2 weeks. If your work requires you to undertake any heavy lifting, such as manual labour or physically supporting others, then I advise you not to return to this type of work for 4 weeks. In most instances, employers may allow you to return to lighter or administrative duties before this time.

Remote working has enabled people to begin working on a laptop from home before their physical recovery is complete. In these circumstances, I would advise you not to consider returning to remote working before 1 week after surgery and carefully assessing whether this is appropriate. Your fit note (which will be non-specific about the type of surgery you have had) will usually cover a two-week period, however, a longer period can be provided by prior arrangement or by contacting you GP practice.

Resuming exercise

I encourage you to remain as mobile as you can immediately after surgery. If you have specific needs or require additional support due to pre-existing conditions that limit your mobility, then the physiotherapy team will work with you to put together a bespoke programme of physical activity.

With respect to exercise, start gradually and begin with low-impact exercises and gradually increase the intensity and duration over time. Walking is an excellent low-impact activity to begin with, as it helps improve cardiovascular fitness and builds stamina. The key is building up your physical activity levels gradually especially if it has been some time since you were last active. For example:

- Week one to two: Add 10 – 15 minutes of physical activity to your daily routines every other day over the next two weeks.
- Weeks three to four: Gradually add in more minutes of activity so that you have 20 – 25 minutes of active time over the course of most days.
- Weeks five and beyond: Add more minutes so that on most days you have a total of 30 minutes of activity.

Listen to your body and pay attention to how your body feels during and after exercise. If you experience pain, dizziness, shortness of breath, or any other discomfort, stop exercising and consult your aftercare team. By about 6 weeks post-surgery, you will feel far more confident to engage in more strenuous exercise. At this point, you can focus on cardiovascular exercises (Activities that get your heart rate up), such as brisk walking, swimming, cycling, or using an elliptical machine. Aim for at least 150 minutes of moderate-intensity aerobic activity per week.

Incorporate strength training to your programme. Building lean muscle mass is essential for maintaining a healthy metabolism. Include resistance exercises, such as weightlifting or bodyweight exercises, to improve strength and tone your body. Start with light weights and gradually increase the intensity as you feel able. Engage in flexibility exercises as stretching exercises can improve flexibility, range of motion, and prevent muscle stiffness. Consider incorporating yoga, Pilates, or basic stretching routines into your exercise regimen.

Whilst exercising, it is important to stay hydrated. Drink plenty of water before, during, and after exercise to stay properly hydrated, especially if you've had procedures like the gastric bypass, which can affect fluid absorption. Follow dietary guidelines and maintain a balanced diet that aligns with the recommendations provided by your aftercare team. Proper nutrition is crucial for fuelling your body and supporting your exercise routine.

Finally, stay consistent and make exercise a regular part of your routine as this is key for long-term success. For people who either do not have access to a gym or don't like the gym environment, it is important to find activities you enjoy and make them a habit. Small consistent changes such as increasing your daily steps by taking the stairs instead of the lift or even parking a distance from work and walking the rest of the way can make a big difference over time.

Going on Holiday or Flying

As a general guideline, most bariatric surgery patients are advised to avoid flying for at least two to six weeks after the procedure. However, this timeline can vary, and it's crucial to consult your surgeon directly to get personalized advice based on your unique situation. Traveling long distances and being seated for extended periods during air travel could pose certain risks, such as blood clots, especially during the early stages of recovery.

Common Challenges during recovery

Whilst pain should usually settle during the first week, it is common for patients to suffer from episodes of aching and discomfort due to increased levels of physical activity and other changes which the body is adapting to. Sometimes pain can be a sign of other issues (which we will cover later), but if you are concerned, it is always safer to contact your aftercare team.

In the first 6 to 8 weeks, it is common for patients to suffer from nausea, vomiting and challenges in taking enough fluids because of the restriction cause by surgery. Consequently, energy levels may be lower than usual as your body adjusts and other symptoms such as dizziness can develop. We sometimes see patients who feel emotionally overwhelmed by the significant changes going on in their bodies and this can be a hindrance to recovery if appropriate support is not sought. Some patients may experience some initial regret (sometimes called 'buyer's remorse) about undergoing surgery in the first few weeks, however this is usually short-lived once the initial phase of recovery is complete. These examples once again highlight the importance of keeping in close contact with the bariatric nurses and dietitians. Early support usually results in a quicker recovery and this topic is covered is much greater detail later.

Energy levels can vary between people. For many, the significant reduction in weight and improved sleeping patterns can result in almost immediate improvements. However, for some, energy levels can be reduced due to restricted nutrition and fluids but may also reflect pre-existing deficiencies such as vitamin B12, vitamin D or iron. If fatigue symptoms persist beyond a few weeks after surgery, it is important to contact your medical team for advice.

Identifying complications

Whilst extensive steps are taken to minimise the small risks of surgery, it is not possible to eliminate these entirely. Whilst some of these problems may be identified during your hospital stay, sometimes complications can happen when you get home.

Before you leave hospital, you will be given several methods of seeking help if you have concerns. These include 24-hours access to the hospital ward, details for the bariatric nursing team during daytime hours, and of course contact details of your surgeon's practice. In the unlikely event that you are unable to make contact through these channels in an emergency, then you can also seek urgent medical care through your local Emergency Department.

The following symptoms may indicate a problem that needs urgent medical attention:

- Severe abdominal pain: Pain and discomfort after bariatric surgery should improve gradually over the first week. Intense or worsening abdominal pain that is not relieved by medication or is accompanied by other symptoms may indicate a significant issue such as internal bleeding, bowel obstruction, or infection.
- Persistent vomiting: If you experience persistent vomiting that lasts for more than a few hours, it could be a sign of a blockage or stricture

in the digestive tract. Accessing medical advice early will ensure that you don't develop dehydration and that the cause can be treated early.

Possible signs of complications in the first month after bariatric surgery

Difficulty breathing
- Pulmonary embolism (PE) – also look out for calf pain!
- Chest infection

Bleeding
- Bleeding from wounds
- Vomiting blood
- Bleeding from back passage

Persistent vomiting
- Bowel obstruction
- Stricture/narrowing
- Stomach Inflammation

Severe Abdominal Pain
- Internal bleeding
- Bowel obstruction
- Infection (leaks)

High temperature
- Infections (wounds, a leak or urinary)
- Internal bleeding

Chest pain
- Heart-related complications
- Pulmonary embolism (PE)
- Chest infection

Irregular or fast heartbeat
- Dehydration
- Heart related complications
- Sepsis

Dizziness
- Dehydration
- Bleeding
- Low blood pressure

Very dark urine
- Dehydration
- Can occur with infection and other complications

- Difficulty breathing: Shortness of breath, rapid breathing, chest pain, or coughing up blood can indicate a pulmonary embolism (or blood

116

clot in the lungs), or another respiratory problem. This is an emergency, and immediate medical attention is necessary.

- Uncontrolled bleeding: If you notice excessive bleeding from your incision site or have significant blood loss through vomiting, bowel movements, or urine, immediate medical attention is required.
- Signs of infection: Redness, swelling, warmth, tenderness, pus, or fever at the surgical site or in other parts of the body can indicate an infection.
- Severe chest pain or irregular heartbeat: Intense or persistent chest pain that is not relieved by rest or medication could indicate a heart-related issue or other serious complication. If you notice a sudden increase in heart rate, palpitations, or an irregular heartbeat, it's important to seek medical attention.
- Significant changes in blood pressure: A sudden drop in blood pressure, light-headedness, or fainting may indicate internal bleeding, dehydration, or other complications. If in doubt, seek medical attention if you experience these symptoms.

Remember that whilst the chances of serious complications are rare, the earlier a problem is identified, the quicker the necessary treatment can be started, and then better the outcome will be in the long run.

Managing Medications After Surgery

One of the key benefits of bariatric surgery is the significant improvement in weight-related medical conditions. As a result, patients often see an immediate reduction in the doses of medications required and, in many cases, patients can stop medication altogether. Careful liaison with your GP and hospital specialist is required, again highlighting the importance of good communication and appropriate planning ahead of surgery.

Bariatric surgery can also change the way that certain medications are handled and absorbed by the body. An understanding of these processes is vitally important to ensure that you remain safe. This highlights the importance of a comprehensive aftercare team that includes specialist bariatric pharmacists who can coordinate this aspect of your care.

Diabetes

Oral diabetic medications such as metformin are usually not required immediately after surgery because of the physiological changes that occur and the significant reduction in oral intake resulting from surgery. Doses of other medications such as insulin will also need to be altered. Close monitoring of your blood sugars is required in this period, and support from your diabetes care team is essential to make sure that blood sugars are not too low or too high. More patients who take insulin are using continuous glucose monitors which makes this process more manageable.

Hypertension medications

For many patients with hypertension, surgery results in an immediate reduction in blood pressure. As a result, blood pressure medications can be either stopped or reduced. Again, close supervision by your GP of blood pressure medications is necessary. A common consequence of not reducing blood pressure medication after bariatric surgery is a feeling of dizziness and light-headedness when you stand up. This could indicate that your blood pressure is too low. If this happens, it is important to seek medical attention, normally through your GP.

Resuming and changing medications stopped before surgery

Most medications can be resumed straight after surgery. The general advice is that if the medication can be crushed, dissolved, or measures less than the size of a 5 pence piece, then it can be safely taken. If this is not the case, then alternatives (sometimes in liquid form or patches for example) will need to be identified until you are able to restart your usual medications, usually around 3-weeks post-surgery. Another consideration relates to modified or extended-release medications. The usual advice is to switch to immediate release tablets to ensure that the full dose is being delivered to the body. The specialist pharmacist will speak to you about these changes prior to your discharge.

Blood thinning medications

Most patients who were asked to stop blood thinning medications will be able to resume these once we are happy that the risk of bleeding is very low (usually a few days after surgery). In cases where patients have been on newer blood thinning medications known as 'direct oral anticoagulants' or DOACs such as apixaban and rivaroxaban, it may be necessary to change these to warfarin. This is because DOACs are absorbed in the lower stomach and first part of the intestine which is no longer possible in the gastric bypass. There are implications to this as warfarin needs close monitoring with regular blood tests.

Other medications

Patients who have stopped other medications such as biologics are safe to resume them following the initial period of healing. Similarly, for those wishing to restart HRT if they opted to stop them before surgery, can do so. A restart date will be discussed so that there is a clear plan.

Contraception

Special mention should be made in relation to the oral contraceptive pill which may become less effective after bariatric surgery. The general advice is to avoid pregnancy in the first year to 18 months after surgery to maximise weight loss and optimise your nutritional levels. We will discuss this in more detail later. The advice is to consider alternative methods of contraception such as injections, implants, barrier methods or intra-uterine devices as an alternative.

Taking anti-acid medications

To reduce the risk of ulceration and acid reflux, most patients will be prescribed an acid reducing agent such as lansoprazole or omeprazole. This is recommended for at least 6 months after surgery and can be continued or stopped in consultation with your aftercare team depending on your symptoms or whether you take any other medication that can increase the risk of ulcers.

Allergies from new medications and supplements

There are well-established recommendations with regards to supplementation and medications that should be taken following bariatric surgery. We will explore these in greater detail later. However, you should be aware that, as with the introduction of any new medication, there is a risk of developing allergic reactions. These may commonly present as a rash or gastrointestinal symptoms such as diarrhoea. If you develop an allergy, then it is advised to stop these and seek medical advice from your aftercare team so that alternatives can be found. In some practices 24-hour pharmacy services are available to help address any potential medication related issues.

Regular Follow-up arrangements

Frequent interaction with your aftercare team is critical to help manage issues after surgery and ensure long-term success. Whilst follow-up arrangements can vary significantly between practices, current UK guidelines recommend aftercare is provided for at least two years. During this time, regular follow-up with team members (including the surgeon, nurse, dietitian, physiotherapist, and psychologist) can occur at different time points and can be tailored to suit your requirements. For example, if you are facing nutritional or psychological challenges, more frequent interactions with the dietitians or psychologists should be arranged.

In general, follow-up tends to be more intensive in the first 6 months as it is usually during this time where patients can struggle. In my practice, I operate an open-door policy, which gives patients reassurance that they can contact the team at any point during their journey. Make sure you understand the frequency and structure of follow-up arrangements as certain aspects, such as the number of sessions with a psychologist, may be limited. In these cases, you may need to finance additional sessions or aftercare out with your agreed package.

Chapter 9: Diet & nutrition after surgery

What is covered in this chapter?

- Progressing through the early post-operative dietary phases
- Macronutrient requirements
- Micronutrients and supplementations

Introduction

While surgery provides a powerful tool for weight loss, it is crucial to recognize that the procedure alone is not a magic solution. Achieving long-term success requires a comprehensive approach that includes significant changes to lifestyle, with diet and nutrition playing a central role. After bariatric surgery, the anatomy and function of the digestive system changes, and this needs a new approach to eating and obtaining nutrients.

The body's ability to absorb certain vitamins, minerals, and other nutrients may also be affected. As a result, people who have undergone bariatric surgery must follow a specialized diet, pay close attention to their nutritional needs, and often include supplements to ensure adequate nutrient intake.

This chapter explores the crucial aspects of diet, nutrition, and supplementation after bariatric surgery. I would say that for most people, this is the most daunting aspect of life after surgery. Perhaps your knowledge of nutrition is limited or the idea of unlearning what you know and approaching diet from a completely different perspective seems overwhelming. At this point I want to reassure you that this chapter serves as an introduction and guide only, and an opportunity to begin understanding *some* of the main concepts that will be repeated regularly throughout your sessions with your dietitian.

As your recovery progresses, you will become more and more familiar with the terms used in this chapter which provides guidance on how to adapt to the post-surgery diet, manage your nutrient requirements, maintain hydration, and make sustainable lifestyle changes. These changes will be supported by a specialist dietitian who will speak to you ahead of surgery about what to expect, provide tailored advice specific to your needs, and guide you as you progress through the different phases of nutritional recovery. By understanding and implementing the necessary nutritional changes, you are more likely to achieve and maintain your weight loss goals, minimize the risk of complications, and enhance quality of life.

The post-surgery diet

The transition from clear liquids through to solid foods is a critical phase. It requires patience, discipline, and a commitment to adopting healthier eating habits. By following the recommended progression of dietary phases and making conscious choices about food selection and portion control, you will lay the foundation for a successful future.

Each of the following phases from liquids, pureed foods, soft food, and then to solid foods can last between 2 to 3 weeks. This means that the time starting to eat solid foods can take between 6-9 weeks. It is common for phases to take longer, or to come across scenarios where you may need to take a step back to a previous phase before making progress again. Different surgeons may prefer to follow different approaches, and so these timelines should be considered as a guide.

Transitioning to free liquids

The initial stage of the post-surgery diet typically involves a progression from a clear liquid diet to full liquids. The clear liquid phase helps the surgical site heal and allows the body to adjust to its new capacity. Clear liquids include broth, and non-carbonated, non-caffeinated drinks. Another way to define liquids is to consider anything which can pass through a sieve. As healing progresses, full liquids (no thicker than milk) are introduced, including protein shakes, pureed soups (with no bits), and skimmed milk.

Introduction of pureed foods

After the full liquids phase, pureed foods become the focus of the diet. Pureed foods have a smooth, blended consistency that is easy to digest. This stage allows the reintroduction of important nutrients while maintaining a gentle transition for the healing digestive system. Examples of pureed foods include mashed vegetables, lean ground meats, smooth porridge, and pureed fruits.

Transitioning from soft to solid foods

As the body adjusts and heals further, softer foods and then solid foods can be gradually reintroduced. However, it is crucial to choose nutrient-dense foods that are easy to digest and make you feel full. Soft, cooked vegetables, lean proteins, and soft fruits are suitable options during this phase. Chewing food thoroughly and eating slowly is essential to prevent discomfort and ensure proper digestion.

Establishing new eating habits

Beyond the specific dietary phases, establishing new eating habits is vital for long-term success after bariatric surgery. This includes practicing portion control, eating small and frequent meals, and focusing on nutrient-dense choices. Mindful eating, listening to hunger and fullness cues, and avoiding distractions while eating can also contribute to healthy eating behaviours. In addition, keeping in close contact with your dietitian is important as they will provide personalized guidance and support in developing a sustainable post-surgery eating plan.

Macronutrient guidelines

Macronutrients are the major nutrients that provide energy for the body and make up a significant portion of the diet. They are required by the body in larger quantities compared to micronutrients. The three main macronutrients are proteins, fats, and carbohydrates. In the next section, we will explore specific macronutrient guidelines to support optimal nutrition after weight loss surgery.

Protein requirements

Protein plays a crucial role in post-surgery nutrition as it promotes wound healing and supporting muscle maintenance and growth. Inadequate protein intake can also contribute to excessive hair loss after surgery. It is recommended to consume high-quality protein sources to meet the increased protein needs after surgery. Lean meats, poultry, fish, eggs, tofu, legumes, and low-fat dairy products are excellent sources of protein. The specific protein intake recommendation may vary depending on individual factors, such as the type of surgery performed and your weight, age, and activity level. However, a general guideline is to consume around 60-80 grams of protein per day for most bariatric surgery patients. Working with your dietitian can help determine an appropriate protein target and provide guidance on including protein-rich foods into meals and snacks.

Fat consumption

While reducing overall fat intake is beneficial for weight loss and cardiac health, consuming some healthy fats is still important. Healthy fat sources include avocados, nuts, seeds, olive oil, and fatty fish rich in omega-3 fatty acids. These fats provide essential nutrients and can help promote a feeling of fullness. It is recommended to moderate fat intake after bariatric surgery, aiming for approximately 20-30% of daily calories. However, it is important to note that the focus should be on healthy fats while minimizing saturated and trans fats found in fried foods, processed snacks, and high-fat meats.

Carbohydrate management

Carbohydrates are an important energy source, but their intake must be managed carefully after bariatric surgery. High-carbohydrate foods, particularly those high in simple sugars, can lead to dumping syndrome, a condition characterized by symptoms like nausea, vomiting, and diarrhoea. Selecting complex carbohydrates that are higher in fibre and lower in sugar is recommended. Whole grains, legumes, fruits, and vegetables are nutritious sources of complex carbohydrates. It is essential to monitor carbohydrate intake and individual tolerance. Generally, a daily intake of 50-100 grams of carbohydrates is a common guideline. However, individual needs may vary, again underpinning the importance of working with your dietitian to determine the appropriate carbohydrate level for optimal weight loss and overall health.

Tracking your macronutrients

Tracking macronutrients provides insight into the overall composition of one's diet and helps identify any imbalances or deficiencies. It allows you to see if you are consuming enough protein to support muscle maintenance and repair, as well as minimise muscle loss during weight loss. It also helps monitor carbohydrate intake to manage blood sugar levels and prevent dumping syndrome. Additionally, tracking fats can help you maintain a healthy balance between essential fatty acids and limit the consumption of unhealthy fats. This is particularly important for those with altered fat absorption after surgery.

There are various methods to track macronutrients, including using smartphone apps, online tools, or keeping a food diary. These tools provide a convenient way to log food intake and calculate the macronutrient content of meals. They also offer insights into total calorie intake, which can be useful for weight management. It's important to note that tracking macronutrients should be done in conjunction with mindful eating practices and paying attention to hunger cues. It should not become an obsessive or restrictive behaviour. The goal is to develop a healthy and sustainable relationship with food while ensuring adequate nutrition.

Counting calories

Tracking overall calorie intake after bariatric surgery can be a helpful tool for weight management and ensuring an appropriate energy intake. However, it is not always necessary for everyone and may depend on individual factors, such as specific weight loss goals, your metabolic rate, and levels of physical activity. The take home message is that it is more important to ensure that your relationship with food is a healthy one rather than becoming an obsessive practice.

Bariatric surgery already creates significant changes in the digestive system, appetite, and metabolism, which often lead to a reduced calorie intake and weight loss. In the initial stages after surgery, focusing on portion control, eating nutrient-dense foods, and following the recommended dietary guidelines is typically sufficient for weight management. Nonetheless, for most people following surgery, calorie intake is usually restricted to between 800 and 1200 calories a day.

As time progresses and weight loss stabilizes, you may find it beneficial to track calories to maintain a healthy balance between energy intake and energy used. Tracking calories can provide a clearer understanding of overall calorie consumption and help identify any potential overeating or under-eating patterns. It's important to be clear however, that calorie counting is not an exact science. While nutrition labels and databases provide valuable information, the actual caloric content of foods can vary due to factors like cooking methods, ripeness, and individual variations in metabolism and digestion.

Additionally, the body's ability to absorb and utilize calories can be influenced by many factors, making it challenging to accurately predict the exact number of calories burned or absorbed from food. Despite these limitations, calorie counting can still offer valuable insights into dietary patterns and serve as a useful tool when combined with mindful eating, portion control, and a focus on overall balanced nutrition.

Micronutrient requirements

Micronutrients refer to essential nutrients that are required by the body in small amounts, but which are still vital for normal physiological functions. These include vitamins and minerals, which play critical roles in various bodily processes, such as energy metabolism, immune function, tissue repair, and overall health maintenance. In the next section, we will explore the importance of micronutrient requirements and the need for supplementation after bariatric surgery.

Importance of vitamins and minerals

Micronutrients, including vitamins (such as vitamins A, D, E and K and B-complex vitamins and vitamin C) and minerals (such as calcium, iron, zinc, magnesium, selenium, copper), are essential for numerous physiological functions in the body. They play crucial roles in metabolism, immune function, cell growth and repair, nerve function, bone health, and many other processes. Most vitamins and minerals are obtained through the diet as the body has a limited ability to produce them on its own. After bariatric surgery, the altered anatomy and reduced food intake can impact the body's ability to absorb and utilize these micronutrients effectively.

Micronutrient deficiencies after bariatric surgery

Several micronutrient deficiencies are common in people who have undergone bariatric surgery. Many of these may have been present before surgery. These deficiencies can occur due to reduced nutrient intake, impaired absorption, and changes in digestion. Some of the most common deficiencies include:

- Calcium and vitamin D: Inadequate absorption of calcium and reduced exposure to sunlight (which is a source of vitamin D) can lead to deficiencies, increasing the risk of bone loss and osteoporosis.
- Iron: Iron deficiency anaemia is common after bariatric surgery, as the stomach's reduced capacity for acid production can impair iron absorption.
- Vitamin B12: Vitamin B12 from the diet needs to bind with a protein called intrinsic factor to be absorbed in the gut. Intrinsic factor is produced by the stomach which is altered by bariatric surgery. Inadequate absorption of B12, can lead to deficiencies that may result in fatigue, neurological issues (such as numbness which can also be made worse by rapid weight loss), and anaemia.
- Folate and other B vitamins: The rearrangement of the digestive system can affect the absorption of folate and other B vitamins, which are essential for red blood cell production and nervous system function.
- Zinc, copper, and selenium: Reduced intake and absorption of these trace minerals can affect immune function, wound healing, cardiac function, and antioxidant defence.
- Vitamin A, E, and K: The malabsorption of fats can impact the absorption of these fat-soluble vitamins, which are important for vision, immune function, blood clotting, and antioxidant protection. As a consequence, deficiencies in these types of vitamins can lead to issues including bruising more easily.

Recommended micronutrient supplements

To prevent and manage micronutrient deficiencies, lifelong supplementation is necessary after bariatric surgery (especially the gastric sleeve and bypass). The specific supplements recommended may vary based on individual needs and surgical procedures. However, common supplements typically include:

- A-Z multivitamins: Comprehensive multivitamin supplements specifically made for bariatric patients are recommended to ensure adequate intake of essential vitamins and minerals.
- Calcium and Vitamin D: Supplementing with calcium citrate and vitamin D is crucial to maintain bone health and prevent deficiencies.

Additional Vitmain D supplementation may be required as people are often deficient in this.

- Iron: Iron supplements (once daily or sometimes twice a day) are commonly prescribed to prevent or treat iron deficiency anaemia. Iron and calcium supplements should be taken 2 hours apart as the combination taken together may reduce iron absorption. Another consideration with regards to iron supplementation is that it is a common cause of constipation. It is therefore especially important to ensure that you are well hydrated and taking in sufficient fibre in your diet to minimise the risk of this.
- Vitamin B12: Regular 3-monthly vitamin B12 injections (or daily oral supplements if injections are not tolerated or possible) are typically recommended. Even if your B12 levels are within the normal range, it is important to continue supplementation to avoid deficiencies.

Supplementation after bariatric surgery

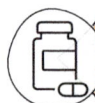

A-Z Multivitamins
- Forceval once daily, or equivalent

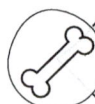

Calcium and Vitamin D
- Adcal D3 twice daily or equivalent

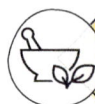

Iron
- Ferrous sulphate, fumarate or gluconate once daily

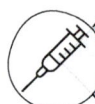

Vitamin B12 injection
- 3-monthly injection (even if levels are normal or high)

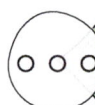

Additional supplements
- If other deficiencies are present

Supplementation should always be taken under the guidance of a healthcare professional or specialist dietitian who can assess individual nutrient needs, monitor levels, and provide appropriate recommendations.

In addition to your multivitamins, it may be necessary to take additional supplementation if deficiencies are identified on your blood tests. All medications and supplements that need to be taken will be clearly described in your discharge document which is sent to your GP.

I am often asked about taking additional supplements to reduce the risk of specific issues such as hair loss or loose skin. These should be taken under the guidance of your dietitian, and whilst by and large these will not be harmful, they must not be prioritised ahead of recommended supplementation.

Blood Monitoring of nutritional status

Current UK guidelines suggest that blood tests, undertaken at regular intervals, are needed to identify the micronutrient deficiencies described above. A full and comprehensive description of what this entails is provided to your GP on discharge from hospital. This is particularly important for those who have undergone the gastric bypass or sleeve gastrectomy. Blood tests should be taken at 3-, 6- and 12-months post-surgery and repeated annually thereafter. The following table provides an example of the key recommended blood tests for the gastric bypass and sleeve gastrectomy:

	3-months	6-months	12-months	Annually
Full blood count	x	x	x	x
Liver function	x	x	x	x
Kidney function	x	x	x	x
Ferritin	x	x	x	x
Folate	x	x	x	x
Vitamin B12	x	x	x	x
Vitamin D	x	x	x	x

	3-months	6-months	12-months	Annually
Parathyroid hormone	x	x	x	x
Calcium	x	x	x	x
Zinc			x	x
Copper			x	x

Hydration and fluid intake

Proper hydration is essential for overall health and well-being, and it becomes even more critical after bariatric surgery. Adequate hydration supports digestion, nutrient absorption, circulation, temperature regulation, and the elimination of waste products. It also helps prevent complications such as dehydration, constipation, gallstones, and kidney stones.

It is important to establish a consistent and mindful approach to fluid intake. The specific fluid requirements may vary based on individual factors such as body weight, activity levels, and any medical conditions. However, a general guideline is to aim for a daily fluid intake of approximately 2 litres or more. This will be difficult to achieve in the first week after surgery but should be the aim by the second week onwards.

After your recovery from surgery is complete, water will be the primary fluid choice as it is calorie-free and essential for hydration. It is recommended to sip water throughout the day rather than consuming large volumes at once. Hydration can also be obtained from other fluids such as herbal tea, sugar-free drinks, and low-calorie electrolyte drinks. However, it is important to avoid high-calorie and carbonated drinks, as they can hinder weight loss efforts and cause discomfort. Remember that all fluids count towards the 2 litres that you need a day, including protein shakes, meal replacement drinks, soup, milk, and protein water. In the early weeks you may be having up to 1.5 litres of protein rich fluids, and the other 0.5 litre from water, tea, and coffee.

To ensure optimal digestion and nutrient absorption, it is recommended to separate fluid intake from meals. Consuming fluids close to mealtime can fill the stomach quickly and potentially lead to discomfort or an inadequate intake of nutrients. It is advisable to wait at least 20 to 30 minutes before and after meals to drink fluids. However, sipping water during meals to aid swallowing and prevent dryness is acceptable.

It is important to be mindful of hydration throughout the day and establish a routine that supports regular fluid intake. Carrying a water bottle, setting reminders, and tracking fluid intake can be helpful strategies in maintaining proper hydration after bariatric surgery. By prioritizing hydration, you can support optimal digestion, absorption, and overall well-being following surgery.

Chapter 10: Nutrition in the long-term

What is covered in this chapter?

- Approaches to supporting nutritional recommendations.
- Sustaining dietary changes in the long-term
- Common digestive changes after surgery

Introduction

After the initial post-surgery phases, it is important to transition to a balanced diet that provides essential nutrients while supporting weight management and overall health. In this next section, we will discuss the long-term dietary guidelines that promote balanced nutrition and sustainable habits after the initial post-surgery phases.

Long-term dietary guidelines

Portion control and meal frequency

Portion control plays a crucial role in maintaining weight loss and preventing overeating. It is important to continue eating smaller meals and paying attention to portion sizes even after the initial post-surgery phases. Consider using smaller plates, bowls, and cutlery to help visually control portion sizes. Additionally, eating more frequent, smaller meals throughout the day can aid in digestion, prevent discomfort, and support steady energy levels.

On the other hand, it is also important not to under-eat which can hinder weight loss efforts, result in loss of muscle mass, and may even lead to weight regain in the long term. Paradoxically, excessively restricting calorie intake can slow down the metabolism and trigger the body's starvation response, making it harder to lose weight and potentially leading to a plateau in weight loss progress. In addition, significant undereating can have detrimental effects on energy levels, mood, and mental clarity. It can result in fatigue, irritability, and difficulty concentrating, impacting on your quality of life and ability to engage in daily activities.

Mindful eating and feeling 'full'

Practicing mindful eating is essential for long-term success after bariatric surgery. Pay attention to hunger cues and feelings of fullness; eat slowly and savour each bite. Take time to chew thoroughly, as this aids digestion and promotes a sense of fullness. Avoid distractions while eating, such as watching TV or using electronic devices, as this can lead to overeating.

The rule of '20' is one example of an approach which can help in this regard. There are different versions of this, however, it can be summarised as follows:

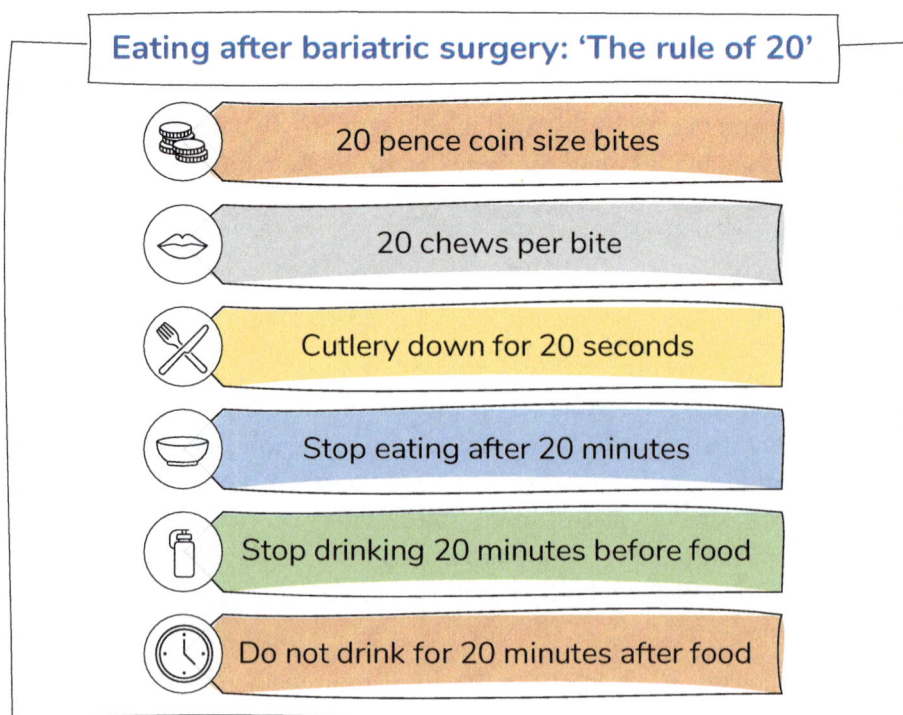

Eating after bariatric surgery: 'The rule of 20'

- 20 pence coin size bites
- 20 chews per bite
- Cutlery down for 20 seconds
- Stop eating after 20 minutes
- Stop drinking 20 minutes before food
- Do not drink for 20 minutes after food

Avoiding problematic or 'caution' foods

Certain foods may be challenging to tolerate or lead to discomfort after bariatric surgery. Carbonated drinks, high-sugar foods, fried and fatty foods may cause issues such as bloating, gas, and dumping syndrome. Whilst an important source of protein and fibre, sometimes tough meats and fibrous vegetables can cause issues and alternatives may need to be found temporarily with the support of your dietitian. It is important to identify and avoid foods that cause discomfort or are not well-tolerated, as individual tolerances may vary. Focus on nutrient-dense, easily digestible options that promote feelings of fullness and overall well-being.

Alcohol and carbonated (fizzy) drinks

By about six months your stomach should have recovered enough to tolerate a small amount of alcohol. But remember, alcohol contains a lot of calories so drinking more than occasional small amounts will mean you will lose less weight. In any case, never exceed the maximum safe limit for health, of 14 units of alcohol spread over a week. Alcohol can also make you hungry, so you are more likely to snack, especially on high calorie foods. Finally, alcohol will be absorbed much more quickly, and blood levels will remain elevated for longer than before your operation so you may feel lightheaded or 'tipsy' on only 1-2 drinks. For these reasons, it is advisable to avoid driving even after a small amount of alcohol.

For similar reasons, carbonated, or fizzy soda drinks should be avoided after surgery. In addition to being devoid of nutritional value, they often contain sugar or sweeteners which can make you feel hungrier. Carbonated drinks can also cause distention of your sleeve or stomach pouch leading to discomfort, bloating, excessive burping and possibly can contribute to stomach dilatation or stretching.

By following these long-term dietary guidelines, you can sustain a balanced, nutritious diet, practice portion control, and incorporate physical activity into your daily routine. These lifestyle habits promote ongoing weight management, support overall health, and enhance the long-term success of bariatric surgery.

Nutritional counselling and support

Role of Specialist Dietitians

By now, you will have understood the need for specialist dietitian support in your weight loss journey; they play a crucial role in providing personalized nutrition guidance and support after bariatric surgery. They help individuals create customised meal plans, educate about portion sizes and food choices, address nutritional deficiencies, and monitor progress. Regular appointments with a registered dietitian are essential for long-term success.

Benefits of support groups and peer networks

Joining support groups and connecting with others (including online forums) who have undergone bariatric surgery provides emotional support, motivation, and a sense of community. Sharing experiences, discussing challenges, and learning from peers can be empowering and helpful in the journey.

Regular Follow-Up and Monitoring

Regular follow-up appointments with healthcare professionals, including the surgical team, nurses and dietitian, are important for monitoring progress, adjusting recommendations, and identifying any concerns or complications. Monitoring blood tests, including micronutrient levels, ensures early detection and management of deficiencies. Current guidelines recommend that blood tests are taken at 3-, 6- and 12-months following surgery and then repeated annually after that. By utilising nutritional counselling, support groups, and regular follow-up, you can have the necessary guidance, accountability, and resources to make informed dietary choices, address nutritional needs, and maintain long-term success after surgery.

Lifestyle Changes and Sustainability

Sustaining some of these nutritional changes can be extremely challenging and I am often asked during follow-up about how best to achieve this. I would generally advise focusing on the following area:

- Prioritise your psychological and emotional well-being: Bariatric surgery not only affects the body but also the mind. Taking care of mental health is important for long-term success. Seek support from mental health professionals, attend counselling sessions, or join support groups to address any emotional challenges.

- Coping with food cravings and emotional eating: Dealing with food cravings and emotional eating can be challenging. Quite often we can mistake head or emotional hunger with stomach hunger. So, try to develop healthy coping strategies such as mindful eating, identifying your emotional triggers, and finding alternative activities to manage stress. In some cases, it may be necessary to seek out additional support from your aftercare team or dedicated clinical psychologists.

- Building a supportive environment: Creating a supportive environment is essential for success. Involve loved ones, educate them about healthy eating, and encourage them to participate in physical activities together. This way you can foster a positive atmosphere that supports healthy habits for everyone.

- Long-term weight maintenance strategies: Maintaining weight loss and a healthy lifestyle requires long-term commitment. Focus on sustainable habits like regular physical activity, balanced eating, continued follow-up with healthcare professionals, and self-monitoring. Celebrate progress and explore different ways to stay motivated along the journey.

- Practical tips: take practical tangible steps to instil healthy eating habits such as only eating at the table, using a small side plate, eating your protein first, removing distractions and temptations, and preparing healthier options such as pick boxes with fruit and vegetables.

By prioritising mental well-being, developing strategies to manage cravings and emotional eating, creating a supportive environment, and adopting sustainable lifestyle changes, you are more likely to achieve lasting success, improve overall health, and maintain weight loss after surgery.

Practical tips to support positive eating habits

Always eat at the table
- not on the go or in the car!

Eat your protein first
- prioritise protein to hit your daily targets

Avoid distractions
- work, televisions, phones

Put tempting foods out of sight
- in a high cupboard

Have a 'pick box' in the fridge
- with cut up fruit and vegetables

How to split your plate after surgery

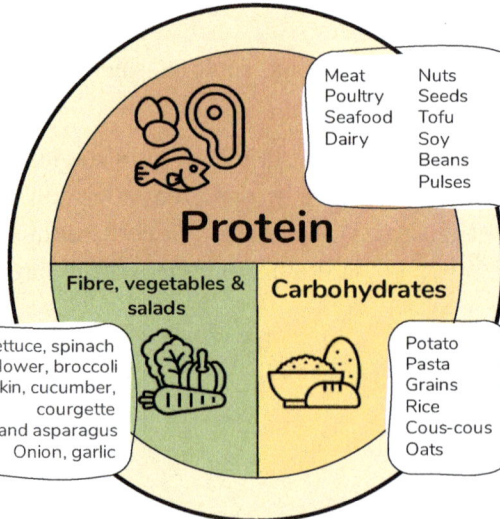

Protein

Meat   Nuts
Poultry   Seeds
Seafood   Tofu
Dairy   Soy
   Beans
   Pulses

Fibre, vegetables & salads

Lettuce, spinach
Cabbage, cauliflower, broccoli
Pumpkin, cucumber, courgette
Celery and asparagus
Onion, garlic

Carbohydrates

Potato
Pasta
Grains
Rice
Cous-cous
Oats

Common digestive changes seen after surgery

Change to taste-buds

Bariatric surgery can sometimes lead to changes in taste perception. These changes may affect how food tastes and can vary from person to person. The following are some common taste-related changes that you may experience after surgery:

- Reduced appetite for certain foods: you may find that your preferences for certain foods changes. Foods that were once enjoyable may no longer be appealing, particularly high-calorie or high-fat foods. This change in taste preference can contribute to a reduced desire for certain types of food.
- Altered perception of sweetness: You may notice a decreased tolerance for sweet foods. This change is often linked to hormonal and physiological changes that occur after surgery. As a result, you may find that previously sweet foods taste overly sweet or even unpleasant.
- Increased sensitivity to bitter flavours: you may also experience an increased sensitivity to bitter tastes. This heightened sensitivity can make bitter foods or medications taste more intense or unpleasant.
- Taste aversions: Certain foods or flavours that were eaten before surgery may become associated with negative experiences, such as discomfort or nausea during the recovery period. Consequently, these associations can lead to aversions and a dislike for specific foods or flavours.
- Changes in taste preferences: Bariatric surgery can result in changes to taste preferences in general. You may develop a preference for different types of foods, such as a greater liking for fruits, vegetables, or lean proteins.

It is important to note that these taste-related changes are subjective and can vary from person to person. While some individuals may experience significant changes in taste perception, others may not notice any changes all. It's advisable to work closely with your dietitian to navigate any taste-related changes and to develop a suitable dietary plan that meets your individual nutritional needs.

Food intolerances

Bariatric surgery, particularly the gastric bypass and sleeve, can lead to changes in the digestive system that may affect how certain foods are tolerated. Examples of these include lactose and gluten intolerances as well as less specific gut changes which can lead to gas, bloating and general abdominal discomfort. There are several reasons why this might occur:

- Reduced stomach size: surgery involves reducing the size of the stomach. This smaller stomach capacity may result in decreased production of digestive enzymes and gastric acid, which are necessary for the proper breakdown and digestion of certain foods. As a result, you may find it challenging to tolerate certain foods, particularly those that are high in fat or require more extensive digestion (such as tough meats, stringy fruit and vegetables and doughy bread).

- Altered transit time: surgery can affect the speed at which food passes through the system. You may experience faster transit time, leading to reduced nutrient absorption and potentially causing digestive issues.

- Changes in the gut micro-organisms: surgery can disrupt the balance of the micro-organisms that normally live within the gut, which can impact the digestion and processing of certain foods. Shifts in the balance of gut micro-organisms may lead to the development of food intolerances or sensitivities.

- Hormonal changes: Bariatric surgery can influence the production and release of gut hormones involved in digestion, such as pancreatic enzymes. Changes in hormonal signalling can affect the digestive process and potentially contribute to food intolerances.

- Individual variations: Finally, each person's response to surgery is unique, and individual factors, such as pre-existing sensitivities or allergies, can influence the development of food intolerances.

It is important to work closely with your dietitian to identify and manage any potential food intolerances. They can provide guidance on an appropriate diet, recommend strategies to manage intolerances, and ensure nutritional needs are met in the context of new or established intolerances. Finally, gut changes or intolerances may not be permanent and can change with time as the digestive tract adapts to its new anatomy. So, whilst there may be foods that you find difficult to manage at the beginning, this may become easier with time.

Summary

Bariatric surgery is by no means a quick fix to reaching and staying at a healthy weight in the long term. Achieving and maintaining optimal nutritional health after bariatric surgery requires dedication, commitment, and a comprehensive approach. By following the guidelines and recommendations provided, you can navigate the post-surgery journey successfully, address nutrient needs, manage weight, and enhance overall well-being.

Remember, it is important to work closely with healthcare professionals, including dietitians, to tailor recommendations to individual needs and monitor progress. Remember to embrace the support of others who have undergone similar experiences and prioritize both physical and mental well-being. By implementing the knowledge and strategies gained from this chapter, you can optimise your nutritional health, leading to a healthier, fulfilling, and transformative post-surgery life.

Chapter 11: Weight loss and weight regain

What is covered in this chapter?

- Phases of weight loss after surgery.
- Expectations related to weight loss.
- Preventing weight regain.

Introduction

A common concern amongst people considering bariatric surgery relates to the amount of weight they are likely to lose and how successful weight loss will remain in the long-term. This is not surprising given the years of yo-yo dieting that most people have been exposed to and that has subsequently been engrained into their psyche. There are several issues related to weight loss that need to be considered and having realistic expectations of what can be achieved with surgery is at the top of this list. In this section, we will explore the patterns of weight loss after surgery and how to protect against weight-regain in the future.

Phases of weight loss after surgery

For most people, weight loss after surgery tends to follow a predictable course, although the patterns within each phase can differ from person to person. Most people will begin their weight loss journey during their liver reducing diet in the weeks leading up to their procedure. Whilst the aim of the LRD is to shrink the liver and allow safer access to the stomach during surgery, people will often lose a significant amount of weight during this period. The LRD also serves as a start point for many to make the necessary dietary adjustments that will need to continue in the longer term after surgery.

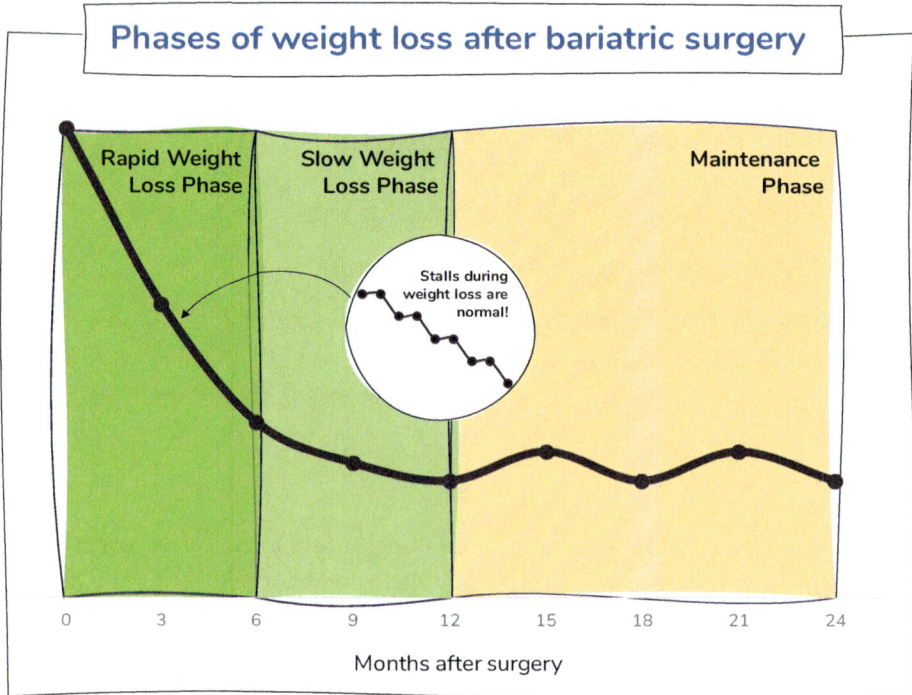

Phases of weight loss after bariatric surgery

Rapid Weight
Loss Phase

Slow Weight
Loss Phase

Maintenance
Phase

Stalls during
weight loss are
normal!

| 0 | 3 | 6 | 9 | 12 | 15 | 18 | 21 | 24 |

Months after surgery

During the initial week after surgery, weight loss tends to be minimal, and mainly occurs because of fluid loss due to the significant restriction that procedures such as the sleeve and the bypass provide. It is therefore very important to maintain your oral fluid intake particularly in the first few weeks to avoid dehydration.

Most weight loss usually happens during a rapid weight loss phase that usually takes place during the first 6 months after surgery. Patients typically experience a decrease in appetite, changes in metabolism, and restricted food intake. Most of the weight loss during this phase is due to fat loss.

A steady weight loss phase usually occurs between 6 and 12 months after surgery where weight loss continues, but at a slower pace compared to the rapid weight loss phase. Patients are gradually adjusting to their new eating patterns and lifestyle changes. Whilst fat loss continues to occur, many people also begin to see significant changes in body composition as they build muscle through increased levels of physical exercise.

144

Weight loss tends to plateau after 12 months (although weight loss can continue for up to 18 months) with the shift in focus moving to maintaining weight rather than further weight loss. It is not unusual to see a slight increase in weight after your lowest point and fluctuations a few pounds either side of a healthier weight range.

Amount of weight loss

As we have previously discussed, there are many factors that contribute to weight loss after surgery, including the need to adopt healthier choices with respect to diet and physical activity levels, and addressing the underlying contributory factors that led to weight gain in the first place. We have also covered how different procedures provide different levels of weight loss (for example the sleeve and the bypass result in much higher levels of weight loss than other options) and we have also explored the impact of other influences such as your start weight, biological factors such as your age and genetics, and whether you are considering first time or revisional surgery.

Speed of weight loss

The rate and pattern of weight loss differs between people following surgery. Most people tend to see the majority of their weight loss during the first 6 to 12 months; however, the process *can* last up to 18 months. It is therefore extremely important to be patient and trust the process. Some people may have rapid initial weight loss compared to others and then plateau, whilst others exhibit a slower and steadier pattern of weight loss over a longer period.

It is also common for most people to see 'stalls' in weight loss which may last 2 or 3 weeks or even longer. Even during these periods, people often notice changes in body composition which are better reflected by using a measuring tape rather than a set of scales. These stalls can sometimes be extremely frustrating and sometimes distressing, and again highlights the importance of keeping in close contact with an experienced aftercare team who can provide important guidance and reassurance.

Losing too much weight

Another concern for some is the possibility of losing too much weight or the fear of 'looking ill'. You should be reassured that losing too much weight is extremely rare. The body has a tightly regulated internal system which knows when to stop losing weight, and as we have learned, weight loss usually stops around 12 months following surgery (by which time the hormonal and physiological changes to metabolism have usually settled). In rare cases where weight loss is excessive, there are usually other accompanying issues and symptoms which point the team to specific causes that may require further attention. Again, this highlights the importance of staying in close contact with your aftercare team so that any problems can be investigated and treated promptly.

Setting a target or 'goal' weight

Goals and targets can be extremely useful in keeping you on track after surgery. However, targets need to be sensible and realistic as they can also lead to unnecessary frustration if they are not achieved. This can overshadow the considerable progress you have achieved so far and have a serious negative impact on motivation and even results in the long-term.

'Goal weights' are sometimes set by looking at the 'ideal' body mass index (BMI). But, as we have covered, BMI is not a necessarily an accurate measure and many people may not be able to achieve a BMI of 25 kg/m² or below. Weight loss in and of itself is but one of many reasons why people consider bariatric surgery. Changes in body composition, improvements in physical and mental health, quality of life and general well-being are as important for most people, and these 'non-scale victories' (NSVs) are key goals that should also be set alongside weight loss. So, whilst setting weight targets can help, it is important to keep these realistic and balance them with other goals you wish to achieve from surgery.

Frequency of 'weigh-ins'

There is no right or wrong answer to this question. What is key here is to strike a balance between monitoring progress and not weighing yourself so often that you become obsessed with minor fluctuations which naturally occur during the process. My advice is to weigh yourself no more than once every 1 to 2 weeks during the initial stages, on the same day and at the same time of day (for example in the morning after waking up and before breakfast).

Many people are also investing in newer weighing scales that link to apps and measure body composition. These can be useful to monitor progress, but you must be careful as the body composition calculations can be inaccurate. As time progresses and your weight begins to stabilise, you should be able to weight yourself less frequently. Remember that it is normal for your weight to fluctuate. Your weight changes depending on the time of day, week and month and you should therefore bear this in mind when choosing when to weigh.

Not losing 'enough' weight

Having realistic expectations of weight loss after surgery is key to keeping a healthy perspective. As we have discussed, surgery is as much about health gain as it is about weight loss and so understanding your non-weight related goals will help keep things in perspective. Remember, if someone's start weight is heavier, then they are likely to lose more weight than someone who has less weight to lose, but they may be less likely to achieve a BMI of 25 kg/m^2 or below. Your age, biology, genetic make-up and many other factors play a role as well the degree to which dietary choices and activity levels change after surgery of course. Finally, keeping in mind what you have achieved so far will for most people help them keep focussed and remove the background noise that can sometimes distract them from the task ahead.

Comparing progress to others

They say that 'comparison is the thief of joy' and this is certainly the case with respect to weight loss. Everyone's set of circumstances and factors that influence weight loss are different. Your journey is your own and assuming that you make the necessary changes, you will give yourself the best change of maximising your weight loss.

Also keep in mind that not everything you see on social media is true and that whilst there are some real benefits to following other people's journeys, there can also be some drawback as well. Remember to keep focussed on your own process, and regularly remind yourself of the achievements that you have made over and above the achievement of others.

Weight regain

The possibility of weight regain, or insufficient weight loss, is one of the biggest fears for people who have undergone bariatric surgery, particularly after many years of yo-yo dieting and seeing years of weight regain after weight loss. However, this topic is often littered with misinformation which needs to be clarified.

Firstly, it is completely normal to regain a small amount of weight after achieving your lowest point after surgery. This is your body settling into its new set weight range. Secondly, remember that whilst bariatric surgery is the single most effective treatment available to help people achieve long term and significant weight loss, it is a tool and does not 'cure' obesity. Obesity is a chronic condition that can relapse over time despite some people's best efforts.

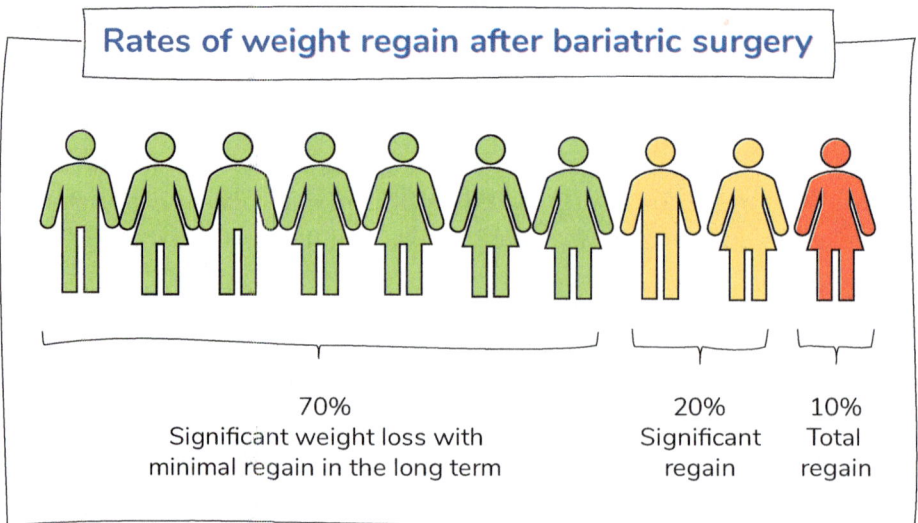

Rates of weight regain after bariatric surgery

70%
Significant weight loss with minimal regain in the long term

20%
Significant regain

10%
Total regain

The amount of weight people regain varies depending on many factors. Based on our best knowledge, if we take ten patients who have undergone surgery, approximately seven patients will lose a significant amount of weight and keep it off in the long term, two will lose and regain a significant amount

148

of weight and one will regain all their weight. This once again highlights the importance of establishing long-term strategies alongside surgery to help control weight.

Preventing weight regain

In order to prevent significant regain, we must understand when and why it happens, and what strategies need to be put in place to reduce the chances of it occurring. Weight regain after surgery is sometimes blamed entirely on a lack of compliance by patients. This is simplistic and relies on the assumption that weight loss and gain is purely a matter of self-control. As we have previously discussed, the reasons for developing obesity are complex, and weight regain after surgery should be viewed no differently. When we explore the reasons for regain in patients, these are a combination of several factors.

Early regain within the first year of surgery is less common due to the significant hormonal changes and restriction provided by weight loss procedures. However, this _can_ occur particularly in the context of continuing to consume high-calorie or processed foods, failing to follow portion control guidelines, or neglecting regular exercise.

Late regain after the first year is more common particularly if there is a decline in motivation, a return to poor eating habits, lack of physical activity, hormonal changes that occur with age, emotional factors, environmental stress, or the development of medical conditions and medications used to treat them. On an individual level, these factors are often the same issues that led to weight gain in the first place, but in some cases, they may be completely new.

Factors related to surgery

In a very small number of cases, there may be factors directly related to previous weight loss surgery that can contribute to weight gain. For example, in the case of a gastric band which is too tight or causing obstruction, the only foods that someone may be able to tolerate are those processed unhealthy foods that melt in your mouth (sometimes known as sliders). As we have discussed, these types of foods result in weight gain and make you feel hungrier. The same situation can arise in the case of a sleeve or a bypass which is causing too much restriction because of a narrowing, stricture, or distorted anatomy.

A common question that we often come across is whether it is possible to stretch a sleeve or stomach pouch. Whilst in principle this can happen, the chances of this being the primary cause of weight regain is in fact uncommon. The stomach is a muscular organ that contracts and relaxes to push food into the intestines. With time, it is completely normal for your sleeve or gastric bypass pouch to relax and for you to feel less restriction. Stretching the stomach pouch takes a significant effort or may be an indication of other problems related to surgery. However, usually there will be other symptoms and signs that your surgeon will be able to identify with targeted questions or further tests.

Strategies to prevent weight regain

The adage 'prevention is better than cure' is no more relevant than it is with respect to weight regain after surgery. It is important to understand that the journey after surgery will, for most people, have its ups and downs. Having a clear understanding of what is expected, will enable you to identify when things are not going to plan. This will most likely occur if you have access to a comprehensive team of experts that can support this process, particularly in the first couple of years.

Having a clear understanding of how weight gain occurs in the first place will give you a roadmap of which triggers and influences you need to avoid. As we have previously discussed, whilst common themes exist between patients, what factors influence your weight are a set of circumstances unique to you. Identify the scenarios which result in poorer food choices and try to avoid these as best as possible. For example, be mindful about sensations of hunger. Genuine hunger occurs gradually after many hours of not eating, whilst head or emotional hunger may occur more suddenly following an advert or feeling sad or bored for example. Understanding these emotions is the first step to halting behaviours that lead to weight regain. We will discuss specific strategies to protect you against some of the challenges which can contribute to regain later.

Managing weight regain

Seeking help early for weight regain is key. It is usually easier to control weight regain from a lower weight rather than starting at a higher weight. Make sure you contact your aftercare team to speak to your dietitians, bariatric nurses and psychologist in the first instance. Identifying the contributory factors (which have been covered extensively already) lies at the heart of addressing regain.

Very few people undergo bariatric surgery without some knowledge of what is required from the perspective of dietary changes and increasing levels of physical activity. Any robust team will have provided education and support both in the run up to and after surgery.

Above all, it is important be honest with yourself about whether changes to nutrition and physical activity levels are being met or whether you need to revisit these. Sometimes wholesale changes are required, perhaps even changes to working patterns or even job types. In some cases, additional psychological support and more extensive therapy may be required if there are mental health factors contributing to negative behaviours.

If you are outside your follow-up package and have regained a significant amount of weight, I would still advise you to get back in touch with your aftercare team. They can often put you back in touch with key members of the team or direct you to health professionals who may specialise in the medical management of weight regain. In some cases, after all factors have been carefully considered, you may be eligible for additional treatments such as injectable medications. And in some cases, after all other routes have been explored, revision surgery may be deemed a possibility.

Summary

Virtually everyone loses a significant amount of weight after surgery. How much weight is lost and whether weight regain occurs and to what degree depends on many factors. Remember that this journey is yours and should not be compared to anyone else's, and that adopting the necessary lifestyle changes in combination with using the support of an experienced aftercare team will help you achieve the best results in the long term.

Chapter 12: Life after surgery

What is covered in this chapter?

- Building habits for long-term success
- Managing emotional and psychological challenges
- Other long-term considerations

Introduction

Bariatric surgery aims to give people back control of their health and quality of life and provides an opportunity to resume a degree of normality often after many years of struggle and trauma. Once you are out of the initial recovery phase, there are several longer-term considerations and challenges that can sometimes arise after surgery. In this section we will cover the main issues to consider and what approaches can be useful in addressing them.

Celebrating Success and Maintaining Motivation

The first 6 to 12 months after surgery are often referred to as the 'honeymoon period' during which most people experience weight loss like never before. Despite this, it is common not to recognise important milestones and accomplishments and focus on what still needs to be achieved, rather than what has been achieved so far. It is essential to maintain a positive mindset throughout your weight loss journey and understand that the process has its ups and downs. Again, this highlights how critical it is to have properly qualified professionals to reach out to at challenging times.

Everyone is different, and strategies for staying motivated and committed to long-term goals will also be different. However, most people benefit from regularly reflecting on their journey to date, realising how far they have come, and celebrating non-scale victories (NSVs). An example of a practical approach to implementing this is to take photographs and measurements prior to surgery so that you have an objective yard stick against which to measure and visualise progress.

Sharing your weight loss journey with others

Undoubtedly, there is still much stigma and misunderstanding about weight loss surgery both in the media and wider society. Many believe it to be a form of 'cheating' or 'an easy way out' (although by now, you will hopefully understand why this is untrue). For this reason, many people undergoing weight loss treatments are nervous about being open about their choices for fear of judgement by those around them. It is easy to say that we should not be influenced by the opinions of those around us, particularly people who have not walked a mile in our shoes, or who will never understand how obesity can affect every aspect of daily life. In the end however, we are only human.

For those that decide to share their journey (whether to a select few or more widely), there are several benefits. People are often surprised by how many of those around them have similar struggles with their weight. Seeing friends or family take the courageous step of seeking medical support can often be the catalyst for others to consider a similar approach. Whilst resources such as this book can help provide a balanced and comprehensive understanding of expectations after surgery, listening to the lived of experience of those who have undergone surgery provides a unique and invaluable perspective. You may have benefitted from reading about other people's experiences on social media yourself.

Finally, I often find that initial criticism from close friends and family towards weight loss surgery can often come from a place of worry about their loves one's safety. Often these concerns completely vanish once the initial period of post-operative recovery is complete, and they begin to see the longer-term positive impacts on physical and mental health. Ultimately, the decision whether to be open about your decision is entirely a personal one which only *you* should decide.

Building Healthy Habits for Long-Term Success

Throughout this book, the importance of behaviour modification and lifestyle changes has been regularly highlighted as a key foundation on which to build long-term success. This includes education about nutrition and diet, but also includes introducing more physical activity. This will naturally be easier to undertake as your weight reduces. Many people think that physical activity means going to the gym, however that is neither necessarily true nor is it a preferred choice for many.

There are lots of approaches to increasing levels of physical activity without going to the gym. These include increasing your daily steps, walking to and from work or parking a distance away and walking the remainder, taking the stairs instead of the lift, and going for a brisk walk during your lunch time to break up the day. All these examples count towards increasing physical activity levels that will help maintain weight loss in the long term. And of course, there is good evidence to suggest that regular physical activity at a lower intensity is far more beneficial than an intense gym session once every blue moon.

Where the gym is particularly useful is in pursuit of building muscle. Muscle helps to increase your metabolic rate by burning energy in the background whilst you go about your day-to-day activities. So, whilst generally improving your activity levels by increasing your daily steps is needed, it is important to incorporate some resistance or weights into your programme. Finally, the gym can be useful in providing a more structured approach to physical activity, especially when signing up for regular classes, which of course also have the added benefit of introducing you to like-minded people.

We've already covered the importance of setting yourself realistic goals with respect to weight loss and how tracking apps can be effective in helping you achieve this. Exercise and physical activity levels should be no different. Long-term success is also heavily reliant on understanding your own journey with obesity, as well as the triggers you need to avoid reducing the risk of weight regain in the future.

Finally, remember the affect that lifestyle changes can have on those around you. The changes you go through after bariatric surgery can have huge impacts on family members, particularly children, who learn behaviours from the actions of those around them more so than through direct verbal instruction. Changing your nutritional habits will undoubtedly impact on improving the health of others in your home. This is an often overlooked, yet important contribution to reducing the risk of obesity and weight-related medical conditions to future generations.

Post-operative challenges

Bariatric surgery can bring about significant physical changes, but there are also several psychological and social challenges that need to be considered. These can affect different people to a greater or lesser degree, but commonly include:

- Adjusting to body image changes: Rapid weight loss can lead to dramatic changes in body shape and size. While these changes are often positive, some individuals may struggle with adjusting to their new appearance and may experience issues with body image.
- Emotional fluctuations: After bariatric surgery, some individuals may experience emotional fluctuations because of hormonal changes and adjusting to a new eating pattern. These fluctuations can include mood swings, depression, anxiety, and irritability. Emotional eating habits may also resurface as a coping mechanism for dealing with these emotions.
- Relationship changes: Significant weight loss can sometimes impact personal relationships. People may receive different reactions from family, friends, and even acquaintances, which can lead to both positive and negative changes in relationships. Adjusting to these dynamics can be challenging.
- Food-related challenges: Surgery involves a change in eating habits and restrictions on the amount and types of food that can be consumed. Following the surgery, you will need adapt to a new way of eating, which can be both physically and emotionally challenging. Some people may experience feelings of deprivation, struggle with portion control, or face difficulties with adhering to dietary guidelines.
- Identity and self-esteem issues: Surgery can sometimes raise questions about personal identity, particularly if an individual's weight played a significant role in their self-perception. Adjusting to a new body and lifestyle may require redefining one's identity, which can impact self-esteem and self-confidence.

- Fear of weight regain: Finally, the fear of regaining weight can be a persistent concern for people who have undergone surgery. This fear may lead to anxiety and an intense focus on weight maintenance, which can affect psychological well-being.

Managing post-operative challenges

To address these challenges, it is necessary to have a support system in place. In addition to an experienced aftercare team, support can also include more specialised mental health professionals, support groups, and loved ones who can provide emotional support, guidance, and understanding throughout the journey. Seeking counselling or therapy can be beneficial in managing these psychological challenges and developing healthy coping strategies. Managing the psychological challenges following bariatric surgery requires a balanced and comprehensive approach that effectively addresses both emotional and behavioural aspects.

The following examples of effective approaches may help you S.H.I.E.L.D. yourself from these challenges:

- **S**upport from other patients: Building a strong support system is crucial. Connect with others who have undergone bariatric surgery, join support groups, or seek out online communities where you can share experiences, receive advice, and find emotional support. Engaging with others who understand your journey can be immensely helpful.
- Developing a **H**ealthy mind through psychological support and therapy: Consider working with a mental health professional who specialises in bariatric surgery or weight management. Therapy can help you navigate the emotional and psychological changes, address body image concerns, cope with stress, develop healthy coping mechanisms, and explore any underlying emotional issues related to food and eating. Cognitive-behavioural therapy (CBT) can be beneficial in addressing the emotional and behavioural aspects of bariatric surgery. CBT helps identify and modify negative thought patterns, develop coping strategies, and improve body image and self-esteem. It can also address issues like emotional eating, stress management, and developing a healthy relationship with food.

Managing emotional and psychological challenges after bariatric surgery

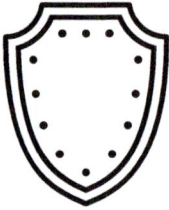

Support from other people & patients

Healthy mind (therapy)

Interact with aftercare

Exercise and physical activity

Learn to self-care

Dietary and nutritional counselling

S.H.I.E.L.D.

- **I**nteract regularly with your aftercare team: Attend all scheduled follow-up appointments with your bariatric surgeon, dietitian, and other healthcare professionals involved in your post-surgery care. They can monitor your progress, address any concerns or challenges, and provide guidance and support along the way.
- **E**xercise and physical activity: Engaging in regular physical activity not only supports weight management but also has a positive impact on mental well-being. Consult with your aftercare team to identify the best exercise options for you, and gradually incorporate physical activity into your routine.
- **L**earn to self-care and manage stress: Prioritize self-care activities that promote relaxation and stress reduction. This can include practices such as meditation, deep breathing exercises, journaling, engaging in hobbies, and finding ways to relax and unwind. Effective stress management can help prevent emotional eating and improve overall well-being.
- **D**ietary and nutritional counselling: Seek guidance from a registered dietitian who specializes in bariatric surgery. They can provide

education and support in adapting to your new dietary requirements, meal planning, portion control, and making healthy food choices. Nutritional counselling can also help address emotional eating patterns and develop a positive relationship with food.

Remember that each person's journey is unique, and it's vital to find the approaches that work best for you. Importantly, be patient with yourself, practice self-compassion, and seek professional help when needed.

Gut changes after surgery

As we have covered, bariatric surgery results in both anatomical and physiological changes to the gastrointestinal tract such as:

- A reduced stomach size.
- Reduced capacity to absorb certain nutrients.
- Challenges with consuming fibre and an adequate volume of fluids.
- Changes to the speed at which food passes through the digestive tract.
- Changes to the balance of the gut micro-environment including the acid/base balance and changes to the bacteria which live in it.
- Changes to hormones and enzymes needed for digestion.

In some people, these alterations can lead to several functional issues that result in:

- Changes to bowel habits (both diarrhoea and constipation).
- Altered levels of restriction.
- Persistent nausea.
- Symptoms such as bloating, burping, stomach rumbling and discomfort.
- Dumping Syndrome.
- Gastro-oesophageal reflux
- And of course, food intolerances which we have already covered.

Not everyone faces these problems, and for the most part, symptoms can be managed by dietary changes. In rare cases additional medical support and treatments may be required. Sometimes these issues may be entirely unrelated to your surgery. Again, this underscores the requirement for accessible aftercare with appropriately qualified healthcare professionals.

Dumping Syndrome

Dumping syndrome is a group of symptoms that can occur particularly after consuming food and drink which are high in refined sugars and carbohydrate. This tends to occur more frequently in those who have undergone gastric bypass surgery more so than the gastric sleeve, but lots of other types of gastrointestinal surgery can also result in dumping. Typically, patients feel unwell and can suffer from:

- Dramatic changes in blood sugar levels (hypoglycaemia)
- Nausea
- Abdominal cramps and pain
- Diarrhoea
- Sweating
- Flushing or redness of the skin
- Rapid heartbeat
- Dizziness or light-headedness

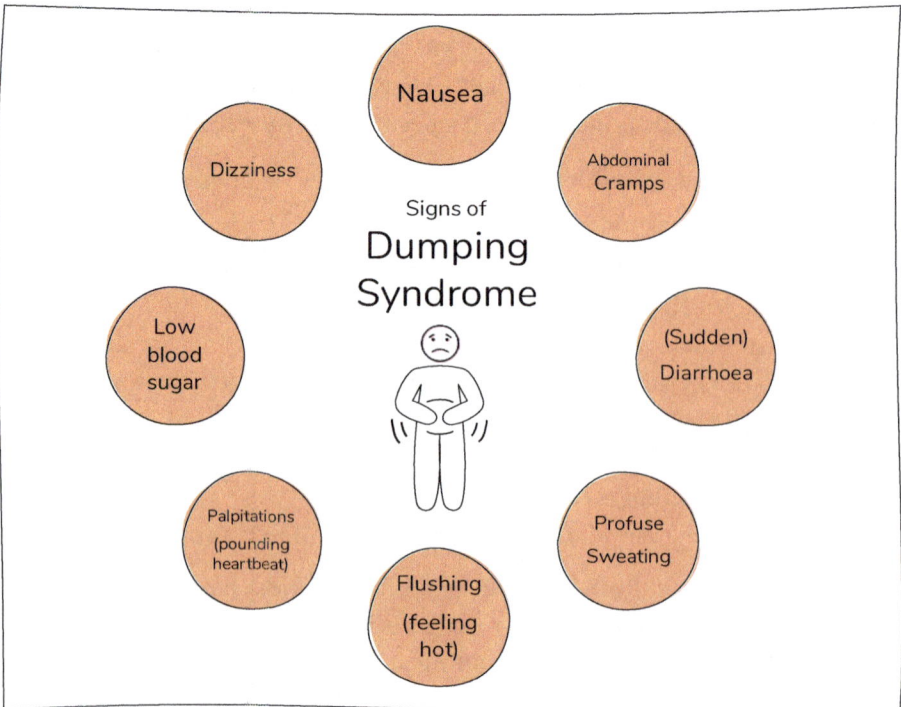

Nausea

Dizziness

Abdominal Cramps

Signs of

Dumping Syndrome

Low blood sugar

(Sudden) Diarrhoea

Palpitations (pounding heartbeat)

Profuse Sweating

Flushing (feeling hot)

Dumping syndrome occurs when food moves too quickly from the stomach to the small intestine. This rapid movement can cause a surge in insulin, which leads to a rapid drop in blood sugar levels (called hypoglycaemia). The symptoms of dumping syndrome can be mild or severe and may occur immediately after eating or several hours later ('early' or 'late' Dumping). In addition, you may not experience all the symptoms described above.

To manage symptoms, people are usually advised to avoid trigger foods, eat small, frequent meals throughout the day, and drink liquids separately from meals. In some cases, medications may be prescribed to help manage symptoms and in extremely rare case where symptoms cannot be controlled, revision surgery to reverse a bypass may be needed.

Gastro-oesophageal reflux (GORD/GERD)

In certain cases, bariatric surgery can lead to the development (or worsening) of reflux symptoms. This occurs when acid and fluid which normally sits within the stomach travels back up into the oesophagus causing a sensation of burning. Symptoms of GORD can be worse in patients who have undergone the gastric balloon, gastric band, and the gastric sleeve more so than the gastric bypass. In the case of the mini-bypass, reflux may be due to bile travelling from the small intestine rather than acid from the stomach. Reflux symptoms can also be made worse by dietary choices and certain medications, so ensuring that these are reviewed is important.

For the most part, GORD symptoms can be managed by taking anti-acid medications (known as proton pump inhibitors or PPIs such as omeprazole or lansoprazole). Current guidance suggests that in the case of the gastric band, sleeve and bypass, a double dose of PPI medication (once in the morning and evening) should be taken for up to six months. This can then be reduced to once daily to keep on top of any remaining symptoms for a further 18 months. For patients who have a gastric balloon, PPI medication should be continued for the duration of the time that the balloon is in the stomach.

Where symptoms are poorly uncontrolled, further investigation may be required in the form of a barium swallow (X-ray) test and a gastroscopy. These may reveal other abnormalities such as narrowing or twists of the stomach, ulcers, a hiatus hernia, or other problems. These tests will help guide any further investigations or treatments that may be required.

Hair Loss

Hair loss is a relatively common response to the stress of surgery, rapid weight loss and certain nutritional deficiencies such as protein, iron, zinc, selenium and biotin. The extent and duration of hair loss varies between individuals, but usually occurs between 3 to 6 months after surgery and is generally considered temporary and self-limiting. That of course does not make It any less distressing. As weight loss stabilises, the body adapts to changes and nutritional levels improve, hair loss will stop and begin to grow back usually around 9-months post-surgery.

The exact mechanisms of hair loss are not fully understood, but it is thought that several factors disrupt the normal hair growth cycle, causing a higher percentage of hair follicles to enter the resting phase and leading to shedding of hair. While it may not be possible to completely prevent hair loss after bariatric surgery, there are steps that can be taken to minimise its impact. These include ensuring adequate fluid and nutrition, particularly protein intake, and taking recommended vitamin and mineral supplements such as iron, zinc, and biotin to prevent deficiencies. Regular follow-up with your aftercare team, such as a dietitian, can help monitor nutrient status and provide guidance on dietary modifications. It is also important to avoid crash diets or extreme calorie restrictions that can exacerbate hair loss.

Loose Skin

Loose skin is a common concern for those who lose a significant amount of weight through surgery. It is difficult to predict exactly how much of an issue this will be for each person as everyone is different. However, there are some known factors which might affect how much of an issue this becomes. These include:

- Age: As we get older, skin becomes less elastic due to reduced collagen.
- The amount of weight loss achieved: The more weight you lose, the more likely you will suffer from loose skin.
- Biology and genetics undoubtedly play a part.
- Smoking: Nicotine products can reduce collagen production, reduce blood flow to tissues and lead to increased skin aging which makes loose skin more probable.

- Skin complexion: Certain skin colour types and excessive sun exposure can result in loose skin.

My usual response to concerns about loose skin is to ask whether the possibility outbalances the benefits of surgery. I have genuinely yet to meet a single person who has been put off by this. While it is not possible to eliminate loose skin after weight loss, a combination of approaches can be used to reduce its impact:

- Gradual and steady weight loss: Losing weight gradually and maintaining a stable weight can allow the skin to adjust slowly, reducing the risk of excessive sagging. Rapid weight loss can increase the likelihood of loose skin which is of course more likely with bariatric surgery.
- Build muscle and tone: Strength training exercises can help build muscle mass, which can provide some natural support to the skin and improve body contour. Focusing on exercises that target the areas where loose skin is most prominent can be particularly beneficial.
- Stay hydrated and moisturise: Proper hydration is essential for skin health and elasticity. Drink an adequate amount of water to keep the skin hydrated. Additionally, regularly moisturize the skin to help improve its appearance and maintain its elasticity.
- Balanced nutrition: Eating a nutrient-rich diet that includes a variety of fruits, vegetables, lean proteins, healthy fats, and whole grains can support skin health. Nutrients like vitamin C, vitamin E, zinc, and protein are particularly important for skin elasticity and collagen production.
- Maintain a healthy lifestyle: Avoid smoking, as it can contribute to skin aging and reduced elasticity. Protect your skin from excessive sun exposure by using sunscreen and wearing protective clothing.
- Consider collagen-boosting supplements: Some supplements, such as collagen peptides or those containing nutrients like biotin and vitamin C, may support skin health and collagen production. However, it is important to consult with a healthcare professional before starting any supplements and not to prioritise these over the multivitamins and supplements recommended after surgery.
- Plastic surgery: In cases of significant loose skin that is causing physical discomfort or negative psychological impacts, surgical

procedures such as body contouring or skin removal surgeries undertaken by specialist plastic surgeons may be an option.

Plastic Surgery

Common areas where plastic surgery after weight loss can be targeted include:

- Abdomen
- Breasts
- Buttocks and lateral thighs
- Face and neck
- Upper arms
- Inner thighs
- Side of chest and back

This is rarely carried out through the NHS and for most is privately funded. Current recommendations are that plastic surgery should only be considered once weight loss has been maximised (ideally BMI less than 30-35) and has stabilised for at least 3 but ideally 6 months. This usually occurs by around 18 to 24 months following bariatric surgery. Finally, if you are considering corrective surgery, my strong advice is to consult a surgeon with a track record of excellent outcomes in patients who have undergone bariatric surgery.

Gallstones

Current research suggests that approximately 1 in 5 people will develop gallstones after bariatric surgery. Gallstones occur when bile produced by the liver, which is usually liquid and stored in the gallbladder, forms tiny crystals and over time grows into stones. Any process which results in rapid weight loss increases your chance of developing gallstones.

They can cause symptoms such as pain and infections which is a strong reason to consider further surgery to remove the gallbladder. Usually at this point, people will have lost a lot of weight, making it more straightforward to undertake than if they had undergone the procedure before weight loss surgery.

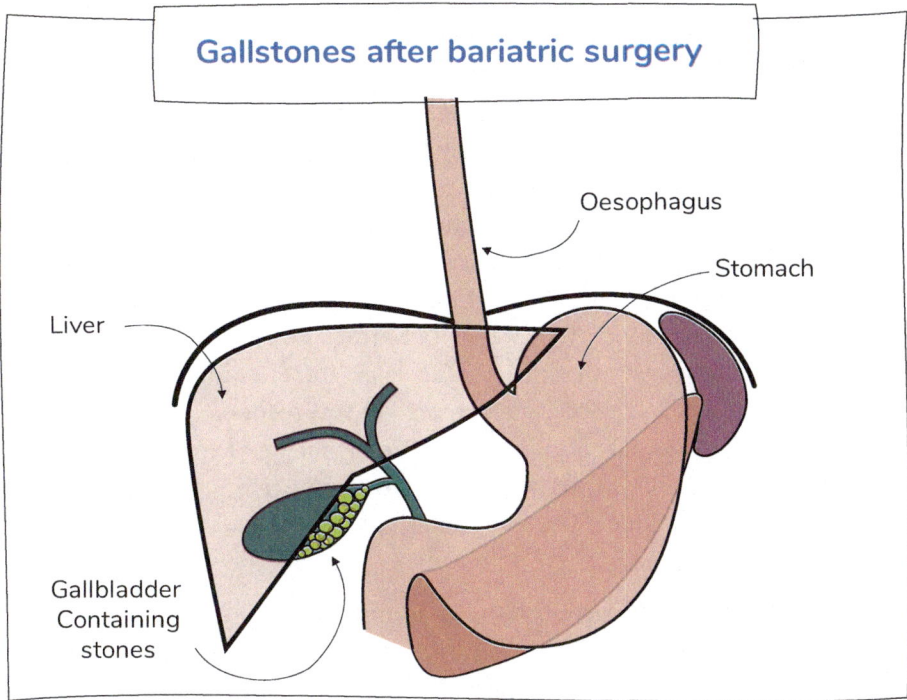

Gallstones after bariatric surgery

Oesophagus

Stomach

Liver

Gallbladder
Containing
stones

Patients commonly ask whether the gallbladder should be removed at the same time as your weight loss surgery. If you already have gallstones that cause you symptoms, then this can certainly be considered. As we have previously discussed, this is not always a straightforward decision, and other factors need to be considered. If you do not have gallstones, the current guidance is not to have the gallbladder removed as this procedure can lead to the risk of complications.

Pregnancy & Family Planning

For many women, improving fertility is an important motivation in pursuing weight loss surgery. The weight loss achieved can often lead to improvement in hormone regulation and increased chances of ovulation. Assuming you are otherwise well, pregnancy is normally safe for both mother and baby after bariatric surgery. However, there are a few key recommendations to consider:

- Current guidelines recommend waiting at least 12 to 18 months after surgery *before* planning a pregnancy, to ensure that weight loss has plateaued and that your nutrient levels are within the normal range. There may also be a slightly increased chance of miscarriage if you fall pregnant too soon, although the research evidence in this area is mixed.
- Close monitoring of your nutritional status is required more regularly than usual to avoid deficiencies *during* pregnancy. You will need to take additional supplementation over and above what would usually be recommended following bariatric surgery. It is therefore important to keep in close contact with the aftercare team who will be able to provide specific guidance in this respect.
- There may be surgery specific factors that need to be considered. For example, if you have a gastric band in place, it may need to be emptied to reduce the possibility of problems such as vomiting during pregnancy.

If you fall pregnant earlier than recommended, then do not worry. Pregnancy can still be safe; however, it is important to inform your aftercare team and GP as early as possible. You may need additional support particularly from a nutritional perspective and more regular assessment of your baby's growth to ensure all milestones are being met.

You should also bear in mind that your weight loss may be impacted if you fall pregnant before the 12-18 month recommended period when weight loss is greatest. Whilst you will be able to continue your journey after baby's birth, the results may not be as predictable.

Summary

Whilst bariatric surgery results in unparalleled levels of weight loss and other significant health-benefits, it may also be come with physical and mental challenges that need to be carefully managed. The importance of having appropriate aftercare to help you develop and tailor approaches to address these issues cannot be understated. However, with the right support, most people can overcome these challenges and get back to the normality that they desire.

Closing thoughts

As you come to the end of this book, I hope that you've gained valuable insights into bariatric surgery and other medical treatments for weight loss. Surgery can be a life-changing option, providing a path to improved health and a better quality of life.

Throughout this guide, we have explored obesity as a complex condition, the different types of bariatric procedures, the preoperative preparation required, and the postoperative care needed for a successful outcome. It is crucial to approach surgery as a collaborative effort between you and your healthcare team. Open and honest communication with your surgeon, dietitian, nurses, psychologists, and other specialists involved in your care is vital to ensure the best possible results. They will provide you with personalized guidance and support, helping you navigate the challenges that may arise during your weight loss journey.

Remember, surgery is not a quick fix and certainly not an easy way out. It is a tool that, when combined with lifestyle changes, can lead to significant and sustainable weight loss. Committing to a nutritious diet, regular physical activity, and adopting healthy habits will be key factors in achieving long-term success.

It is essential to have realistic expectations and whilst it is extremely safe, understand that bariatric surgery is not without risks. Educating yourself about the team providing your care, the procedure, its potential benefits, and potential complications is crucial. By doing so, you can make an informed decision about whether bariatric surgery is the right choice for you.

Finally, surround yourself with a strong support system. Family, friends, and support groups can provide the emotional support and encouragement needed throughout your weight loss journey. Remember, surgery is just the beginning of your new chapter—a tool to assist you in reaching your goals. Embrace the changes, commit to a healthier lifestyle, and work closely with your healthcare team. With dedication and perseverance, you can achieve a healthier, happier future.

Printed in Great Britain
by Amazon

35312621R00099